A Journey with Hydrotherapy

A JOURNEY WITH
Hydrotherapy

Within a Lifestyle of Natural Living & Natural Healing

GERARD MIFSUD

**Nature Cure Practitioner
Hydrotherapist**

Published by the Power Writers Publishing Group in 2026.

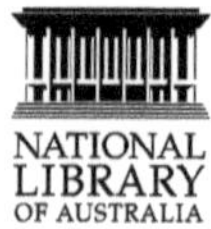

A catalogue record for this book is available from the National Library of Australia

ISBN: 9781764276122

Cover by Andrew Davies.

Internal layout by Andrew Davies.

Disclaimer

Any opinions expressed in this work are exclusively those of the author and are not necessarily the views held or endorsed by others quoted throughout. All of the information, and concepts contained within the publication are intended for general information only. The author does not take any responsibility for any choices that any individual or organization may make with this information in the business, personal, financial, familial or other areas of life.

Profits from the sale of this book go towards the establishment, archiving and dissemination of the Kenneth S. Jaffrey Memorial Library.

The purpose for this publication is to make the simple science, practice, history and application of hydrotherapy within the context of Natural Living and Natural Healing (known as Nature Cure), accessible to all humanity.

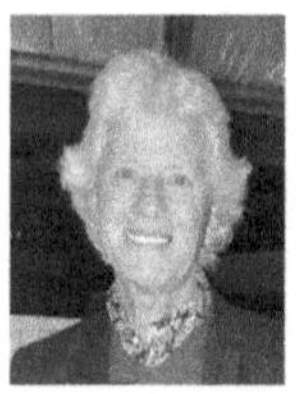

Kevin D. Hinton

Dedication

This book is dedicated to my teacher and dear friend, **Kevin D. Hinton M.A., N.D.** (7 October 1945 – 30 December 2017)

Kevin and I first met at a class he and his wife, Katy Hinton, were running at the local technical college in Townsville. From our very first conversation, I felt I had encountered someone special. That meeting marked the beginning of a thirty-two-year friendship – years of learning, inquiry, and shared exploration across science, history, philosophy, and communication, all within the broader context of natural living and humanity's place in this remarkable cosmos. We became, in the truest sense, brothers and fellow seekers of truth.

Kevin excelled in whatever he applied his focused energy to, particularly in publishing and conveying the teachings of his own mentor, **Mr Kenneth S. Jaffrey**, along with those of other great thinkers in the field of Nature Cure. One of his many remarkable achievements was his embrace of social media as a modern educational platform. Alongside **Angus Holliday**, Kevin helped establish the **Nature Cure Facebook Group**, which quickly grew into a global community of more than twelve and a half thousand health and truth seekers. It became a modern-day forum for sharing the enduring principles of Natural Living and Natural Healing, and Kevin being the consummate educator took great joy in the thoughtful dialogue it inspired – something witnessed firsthand.

Among Kevin's many accomplishments:

- Studied for twenty years under Mr Kenneth S. Jaffrey and received a Doctor of Naturopathy (N.D.)

- Ran a successful clinical practice with Katy for over thirty years in Townsville

- Instrumental in establishing the Townsville Natural Health Group

- Contributed regular articles to the *Townsville Bulletin* local newspaper

- Held a regular community radio spot with interviews on matter of Health

- Co-authored *A Lifestyle for Health & Happiness*

- Trained and mentored more than five students

- Built the Nature Cure Facebook Group to over twelve and a half thousand members within five years — a living archive of knowledge that remains available today

The following extract was written by Kevin Hinton on the ninth November 2011 and is taken directly from the Nature Cure Facebook Group page:

This is an educational site.

I am Kevin Hinton – a Health Educator and the administrator of this site. I studied for 20 years with Mr. Kenneth S. Jaffrey – undoubtedly one of the foremost – if not the foremost Nature Cure practitioner of the 20th C.

I have over 35 years of clinical practice and published "A Lifestyle for Health and Happiness"

We teach the principles and practice of Pure Nature Cure.

We base our teachings on the Art and Science of Nature Cure using Dialectical methods. This means that we base our teachings on natural principles / laws = we are DIALECTICAL MATERIALISTS.

We DO NOT subscribe to 'powers' that exist outside of the material world – therefore we do not and will not discuss religions, spirituality, souls, Gods or any other 'IDEALISTIC' matter.

Please feel comfortable asking questions. I will respond with answers and supporting materials – but please do not attempt to disprove, denigrate or downplay the philosophy and practice of Nature Cure as any such posts will be dealt with immediately by the touch of a 'delete.'

This is posted with all the respect I can muster – thank you for your considerations."

From this social media group Kevin found a small number of dedicated students who, together with myself, undertook formal studies in 2014 and 2015 in the art and science of natural living and natural healing.

Kevin has left behind a legacy that stands as both a gift and a responsibility. It is a vision of health that, if embraced, could shape the future of humanity. We now stand on his shoulders, alongside the health educators of the past two centuries, inheritors of a tradition entrusted to all of us.

Gerard Mifsud, NCP
Hydrotherapist

Contents

Foreword

In my view, an updated and modern 'how to' book on hydrotherapy is long overdue. The practice of hydrotherapy is hundreds of years old, and its efficacy has been tried and proven throughout the ages. However, it has sadly fallen out of vogue with most natural health practitioners and is now almost solely practiced in the domain of Nature Cure.

My teachers Kevin and Katy Hinton introduced me to Gerard Mifsud a number of years ago, and a deep friendship that flowed from our mutual interest and personal practice of Nature Cure quickly developed. Gerard holds a profound understanding of the philosophy and principles of Nature Cure with a particular interest and expertise in the domain of hydrotherapy. He has applied these practices to himself and of course reaped the rewards.

Like so many of us in the field of Nature Cure, Gerard holds a strong desire to share his knowledge to help those interested in applying the principles of natural living and natural healing to improve their health. In writing this book, Gerard has played a major part in ensuring that the knowledge of this time-honoured practice is kept alive in perpetuity.

Hydrotherapy is the only truly drugless and safe method that can be applied to those in the chronic state. As Gerard has outlined throughout this book, Hydrotherapy is best used under the guidance of a qualified health practitioner or Hydrotherapist.

All the best to your health.

Victoria Mohren NCP BOM Acc B Bus.

Introduction

"Life in us is like the water in a river."
Henry David Thoreau

Tell them what you're going to tell them – tell them – then tell them what you told them.

These were the words of my teacher, Kevin Hinton. He would often remind us that true learning comes from applying knowledge, not simply hearing it. His advice has remained with me ever since.

I still recall my first appointment with Kevin and his wife Katy at their practice in West End, Townsville. It was 1985, and I had gone for a complete health diagnosis. A few years earlier I had been in a serious motorbike accident, sustaining compressed discs in my neck and lower back. I was introduced to hydrotherapy for the very first time during that consultation.

Kevin prescribed a comprehensive health-building lifestyle plan for me. It included spinal baths, hip baths, back and neck compresses, and mild inversion. These practices of salvation became part of my daily routine and, when needed, they still are to this day. The alternatives of pain medication and surgery were never an option, especially after witnessing the devastating consequences of spinal surgery endured by my brother.

This book will take you on a journey through hydrotherapy – its meaning, its history, its science, and its application. In Chapter One, you'll develop a clear understanding of what hydrotherapy is. Chapter Two explores its fascinating history, from its modern-day origins in the 1820s as *The Water Cure*, to its use by ancient civilisations.

In Chapter Three, we look at the simple scientific principles of physics, biology, and chemistry that underpin hydrotherapy. This is where you'll get an understanding of what happens physiologically in the body when water is used to restore balance, equalise circulation, and ease pain.

Chapter Four covers the most common hydrotherapeutic applications and processes. Whether you are managing chronic disease, recovering from injury, or simply seeking to maintain your health, these methods offer a gentle, effective, and natural alternative.

Along the way, I'll share my own experiences including the treatments I've used, the results I've seen, and the important dos and don'ts that will make it easier for you to get the most out of the time you put into reading this book. This is especially the case in Chapter Five where I share my experience of using hydrotherapy to handle an unfortunate vehicle crash I had as I was getting ready to hand this book over to the editor.

Finally, in Chapter Six you'll be reading about the position of hydrotherapy within the broader framework of natural living and natural healing, honouring its place as one of the essential tools in the nature cure practitioner's toolbox.

You'll notice that I use images throughout the book to enhance your experience of reading it.

You will come across links to access audio recordings that offer a deeper exploration of the material you are reading only available in the e-book

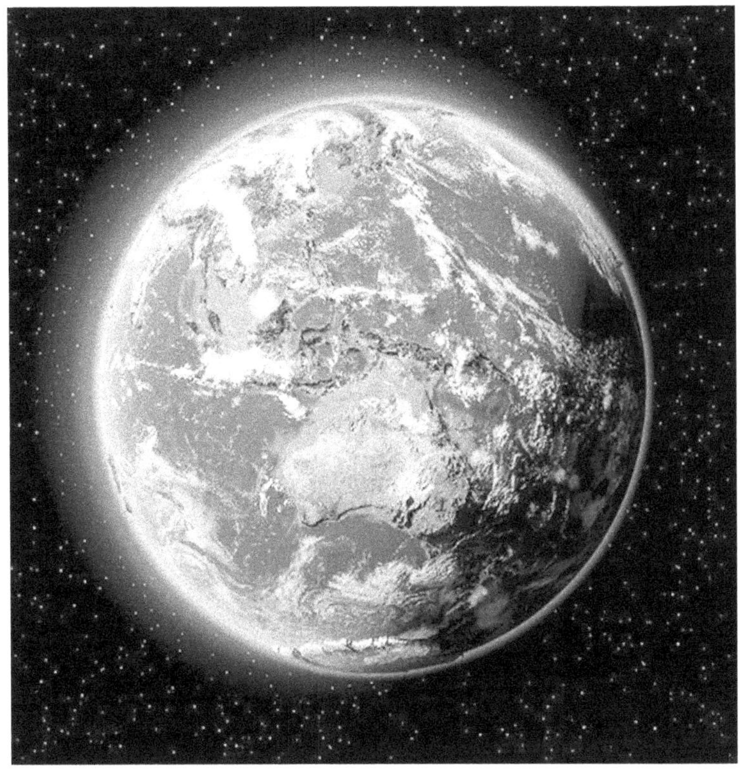

The blue planet – our home

*"Water is the lifeblood that flows through
the veins of Mother Earth"*
Evelyn Parkin – Quandamooka Elder – Minjerribah
(Nth Stradbroke Island) Queensland, Australia

The thing is that we've all experienced water's capacity to bring relief to our bodies, whether we're aware of it or not. A shower or bath, a dip in a cool stream, river, lake, or the ocean. Whether it's in the morning after a night's rest, or at the end of a long day's work, there is nothing quite like the refreshment and invigoration of immersing ourselves in water.

This is no coincidence. I say that because our bodies are composed of more than 60% fluids, and 71% of our planet is covered by water. Science tells us that organic life originated in water. This is a fact that's reflected in the beginnings of human life and birth itself.

The philosophy of natural living and natural healing – what we call Nature Cure – rests on a few timeless foundations. They are:

- To identify and remove all causes of disease.
- To provide the biological requirements for health: sunlight, air, water, living foods, exercise, rest, mental poise, and spinal integrity.
- To allow the body to rest physically, digestively, and mentally when it enters a natural healing cycle.
- To accept that when it is left uninterrupted, the body heals itself naturally and safely.

All forms of life, including humans, are self-regulating, self-reproducing, and self-healing when the correct biological conditions are present. However, it is important to remember that water itself has no healing power. The true healing power lies within your body via its vitality and capacity to restore itself to health. Water is simply the essential medium that assists in this process when the conditions are right.

Many excellent books (see References, page 67) have been written on the efficacy of hydrotherapy. Yet most of these works are no longer easily accessible to the average reader, and they often lack one critical element – the practical how-to details. That is what I hope this handbook will provide.

Aside from my own personal experiences that I share with you in the chapters that follow, there is nothing new in this book. The knowledge presented here has long been published in many earlier works. Yet when I ask people what the term hydrotherapy means to them, the usual reply is – "Isn't that exercising in a heated pool?" To me, this shows just how far this simple yet powerful healing art has slipped from public memory since the golden era of the 1850s. Too often these pools are so heavily chlorinated that inhaling the fumes is unpleasant enough to negate any benefit. Hydrotherapy, in its simplest form, can feel almost magical to the newcomer. Yet our forebears knew it as common sense – an instinctive first response to pain, injury, or illness. The truth of it is that for millennia, the therapeutic application of water has served humanity as a safe, reliable, and effective aid to healing.

Meanwhile, when we're faced with pain and illness these days, we are usually offered pharmaceuticals, creams, potions, surgery, or manipulations – each with negative side effects and uncertain outcomes. I chose another path: to take responsibility for my own health. And so, congratulations to you, the reader, for tapping into a resource that I trust will guide you on your own journey to recovery and vitality. After all, isn't it the best of health that we all truly seek?

Finally, if you decide to use hydrotherapy, I strongly recommend beginning under the guidance of a qualified Nature Cure practitioner. They can design a program tailored to your unique condition, ensuring the correct applications from the very beginning, helping you to achieve faster and more lasting results.

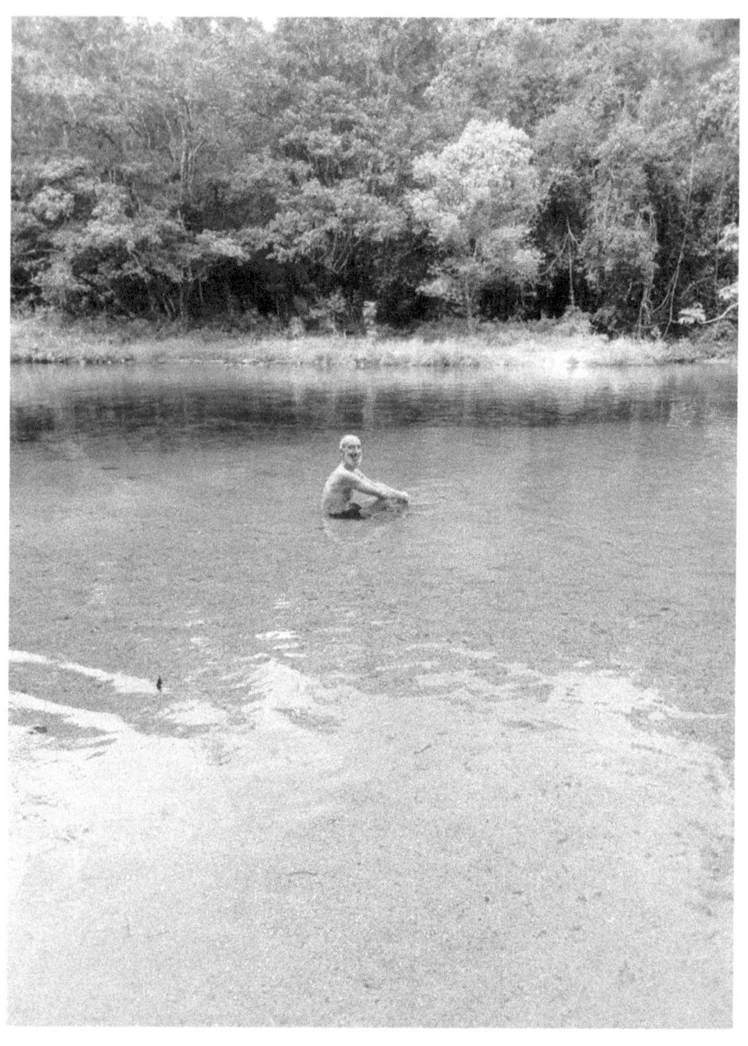

Chapter One

What is Hydrotherapy and Its Purpose?

*"There is no healing power outside the organism, and if
there were, it would be cold water applied judiciously."*
Dr Henry Lindlahr

Let's start with the basics in terms of the meanings of the words that comprise the broader term of hydrotherapy. Hydro = Water and Therapy = Cure. Historically, the word hydrotherapy comes from two Greek words: *hudor* (water) and *therapein* (to heal). Put simply, it means healing through water. Hydrotherapy is the application of water at different temperatures to produce a therapeutic effect on the body. It is a natural way of supporting the return to normal function and balance. In other words, hydrotherapy's ultimate purpose is to help the body restore its own equilibrium. My teacher, Kevin Hinton, would often ask me, "So, young fella, what's the purpose of hydrotherapy?" The answer he expected, which still applies today, is simple: it's to equalise the circulation of blood, lymph, and nerve force within the body.

Many people wonder how water can possibly heal a body that is either sick or injured. The truth is that it doesn't. The real power to heal lies in the body's living vitality. It's our body's innate response to the application of water (whether hot or cold) that produces the conditions for healing to take place. The thing is that health depends on free and balanced circulation. It's only when this is the case, that every organ receives the proper nourishment that's required to perform its functions. When the systems of the body work in harmony, nutrients are absorbed, metabolism is carried out, and toxic by-products are effectively eliminated.

Hydrotherapy in the Nature Cure Philosophy

In Nature Cure, chronic disease is understood as a state of Toxemia in the form of impurities in the blood and tissues that disrupt circulation. Hydrotherapy doesn't supply healing power; it acts as a catalyst, stimulating the circulation and drainage necessary for recovery.

That is why I often repeat the phrase: there is no healing power in water itself. What's more, salts, oils, milk baths, and the like, may feel pleasant, but they are not required to generate healing because they lack the efficacy hydrotherapy delivers. In fact, they are little more than window dressing. If these kinds of extras uplift you, by all means use them, but don't expect any meaningful therapeutic effects from doing so.

Hydrotherapy is both a science and an art. Treatments must be suited to the vitality of each person and their ability to respond. Paying attention to how your body reacts to each application is critical, because your own vitality dictates the outcome.

How Water Balances the Body

The practical effects of water therapy are direct and measurable. Applied with purpose, hydrotherapy can:

- Regulate and balance body temperature
- Increase blood flow to targeted areas
- Improve drainage from congested tissues
- Wash away impurities from the surface of the body
- Tone weak or flaccid tissues
- Relax spasms and pain, helping the body return to its normal function.

The Principle of Quantity and Quality

There is no magic bullet or instant cure in the realm of Nature

Cure. True healing is progressive and depends on restoring natural conditions. One principle applies again and again within this approach to both the healing and maintenance of our body. The principle I'm referring to here is that, 'with an increase in quantity, there will come a sudden and dramatic change in quality'.

This means that repeated, consistent improvements, whether they're achieved through hydrotherapy or lifestyle adjustments, will eventually tip the balance, leading to remarkable change. Don't expect one or two treatments to erase years of poor living habits though. What you will find is that over time with consistency and persistence, the results will be undeniable.

The same principle also works in reverse. Ignore the natural laws for long enough, and the body will eventually reveal chronic disease, often with sudden intensity. I have lived through this process myself and can assure you that patience and persistence always pay off.

The Question of Time

If you have driven yourself hard and fast and now find yourself facing diseases of one kind or other, you may be inclined to ask: how long will it take to recover? The answer is: as long as it takes.

Recovery depends on your vitality, your environment, and your willingness to change your lifestyle. Unlike conventional medicine, Nature Cure does not treat isolated symptoms. Instead, it removes the causes of disease, provides the body with what it biologically requires, and allows the natural healing process, (which is often expressed through fever) to eliminate accumulated toxins.

When fever arises, it is a signal that the body is liquefying and removing waste. At that moment, rest is essential – physically, digestively, and mentally. This process, though sometimes challenging, is the path toward lasting health and vitality.

The True Purpose of Hydrotherapy

To summarise, hydrotherapy is not a cure in itself – but a supportive tool. Its purpose is to aid the free flow of blood, lymph, and nerve force, thereby equalising circulation throughout the body.

When this balance is restored, the body's own healing intelligence can function unhindered. That is the true value of hydrotherapy. It is a simple, natural, and profoundly effective way of assisting the body back to its inherent state of health.

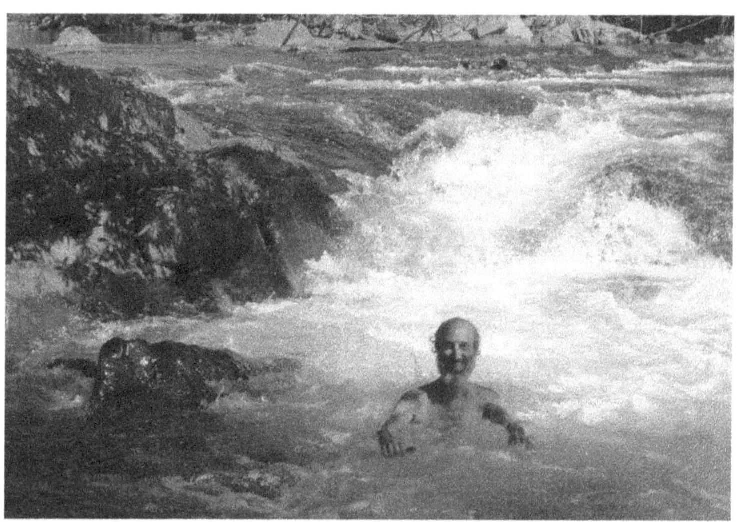

Chapter Two

The History of Hydrotherapy

"In order to understand a thing – you must know its history."
Kevin D Hinton, MA ND and Kenneth S. Jaffrey, ND DC

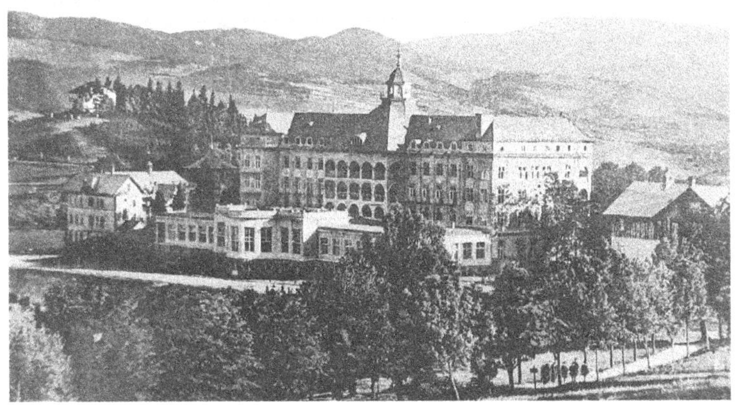

Priessnitz Sanatorium – Jessnik Grafenberg c. 1920

Hydrotherapy is not a modern invention. Its use reaches back to ancient civilisations: Egyptian royalty (2686–1213 BC) bathed in fragrant waters, Hippocrates (460–375 BC) prescribed spring baths to restore balance through *'vis medicatrix naturae'* (the healing power of nature), the Romans built grand public bathhouses, and in Japan, hot springs (*onsen*) became central to cultural health practices.

The modern revival of hydrotherapy, however, begins in 19th-century Europe, with Vincent Priessnitz (1799–1852), a self-taught farmer from Gräfenberg, Germany. Inspired by nature and his own healing experience using cold-water compresses, Priessnitz founded a sanatorium and became known worldwide for "The Water Cure." His methods attracted peasants and royalty alike, setting the foundation for modern naturopathy.

Priessnitz's work inspired others: Captain Claridge (1797–1857) introduced his methods to England; Father Sebastian Kneipp (1821–1897) linked European nature cure with American naturopathy; Theodor Hahn (1824–1883) advocated vegetarianism alongside water cures; and Louis Kuhne (1835–1901) developed new methods like the friction sitz bath and wrote *The New Science of Healing*.

Other pioneers contributed significantly: Frederick Bilz (1842–1922) popularised natural healing with widely read books; Adolf Just (1859–1936) emphasised "returning to nature"; and in America, Joel Shew (1816–1855) and Russell T. Trall (1812–1877) spread Priessnitz's ideas, influencing John Harvey Kellogg (1852–1943), who authored *Rational Hydrotherapy*. John Henry Tilden (1850–1940) further advanced natural philosophy with his seminal book *Toxemia Explained* (1926).

The German priest Benedict Lust (1872–1945), known as the "Father of American Naturopathy," brought Kneipp's teachings to the United States, combining them with Ayurveda and Yoga. Meanwhile, Henry Lindlahr (1862–1924) integrated diet, sun, fresh air, and exercise into systematic naturopathic practice.

In Britain, James C. Thompson (1887–1960) and his son Leslie C. Thompson (1919–1992) carried the torch through the Kingston Clinic in Scotland, while in India, Sarma K. Lakshman (1879–1965) adapted Kuhne's teachings into a distinctly Indian approach, building sanatoriums and emphasising self-treatment.

The 20th century brought further scientific refinement. Professor Edmond Bordeaux Székely (1905–1979) advanced naturopathy with his system of "Cosmotherapy," grounding it in science and mathematics. His influence extended worldwide, including the work done by Kenneth S. Jaffrey (1909–1998) in Australia, who synthesized two centuries of teachings into accessible books and trained future generations.

In Australia, early figures like Dr Otto Abramowski (1852–1910), and later Frederick George Roberts (1892–1977), spread natural healing in Australia. Leslie Owen Bailey (1890–1964) founded the Natural Health Society of Australia, ensuring these traditions continued.

This lineage shows hydrotherapy as a continuous thread, shaped by individuals who observed nature, trusted the body's capacity to heal, and created institutions that preserved this knowledge for us today.

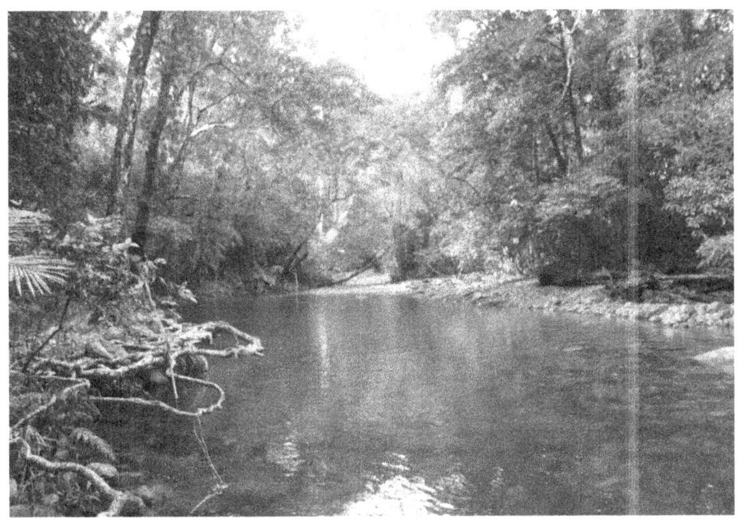

Timeline of Key Figures in Hydrotherapy & Nature Cure

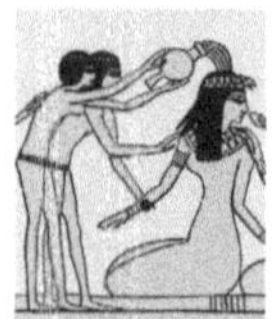

Egyptian Royalty
2686–1213 BC
Ritual and medicinal baths with oils and flowers

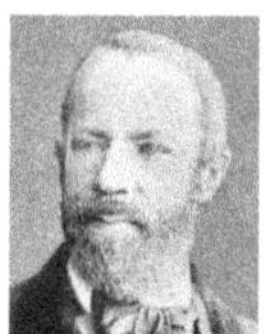

Theodor Hahn
1824–1883
Advocated water cure with a vegetarian diet

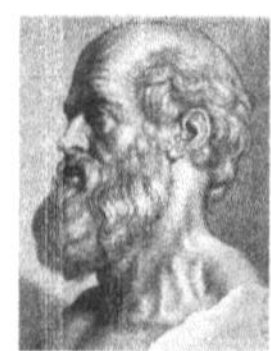

Hippocrates
460–375 BC
Prescribed spring baths; "healing power of nature"

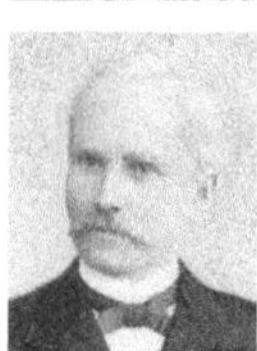

Louis Kuhne
1835–1901
Author of *The New Science of Healing*, invented friction sitz bath

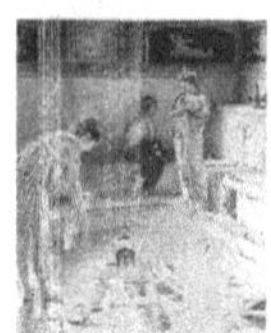

Romans
~500 BC–476 AD
Public bathhouses for health and social life

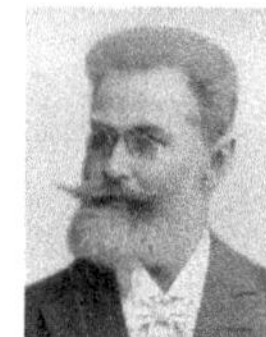

Frederick Bilz
1842–1922
Wrote popular books, established hydropathic institutions

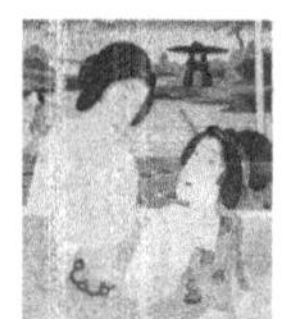

Japanese culture
Centuries-long
Hot springs (*onsen*) for healing and relaxation

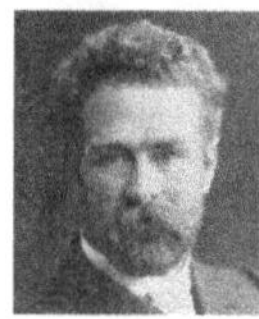

Adolf Just
1859–1936
Author of *Return to Nature*, emphasized earth connection

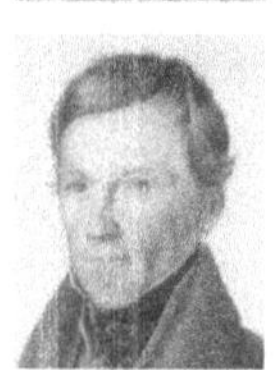

Vincent Priessnitz
1799–1852
Founder of modern-day hydrotherapy, "The Water Cure"

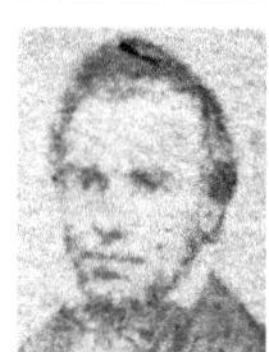

Joel Shew
1816–1855
Early U.S. proponent of water cure, started the Hydropathy Institute

Captain R.T. Claridge
1797–1857
Spread Priessnitz's system to England

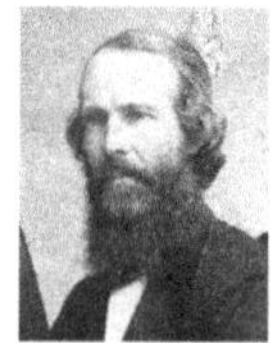

Dr Russell Thacher Trall
1812–1877
Published *The Hydropathic Encyclopedia*, and influenced Kellogg, Founded the Water Cure Institution

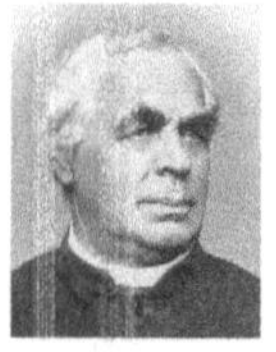

Father Sebastian Kneipp
1821–1897
Linked European water cure with U.S. naturopathy

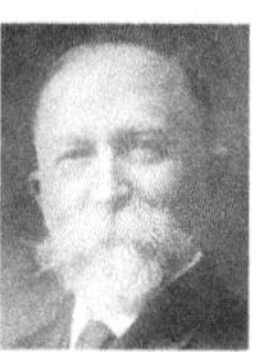

John Harvey Kellogg
1852–1943
Wrote *Rational Hydrotherapy*

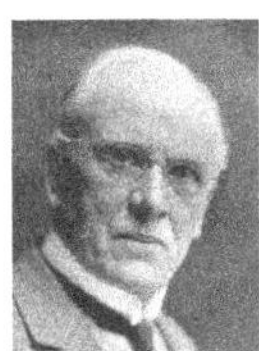

John Henry Tilden M.D.
1850–1940
Author of *Toxemia Explained*

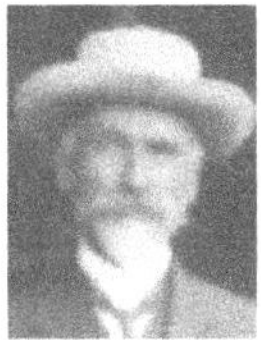

Dr. Otto Abramowski
1852–1910
First naturopath in Australia; founded The Sun Sanitarium

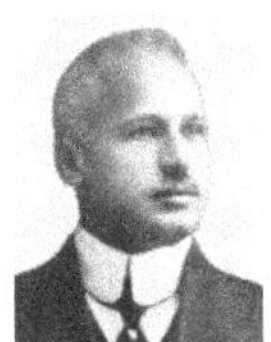

Benedict Lust
1872–1945
Father of U.S. naturopathy, blended the Kneipp cure with Ayurveda & Yoga

Frederick George Roberts
1892–1977
Promoter of natural healing in Australia

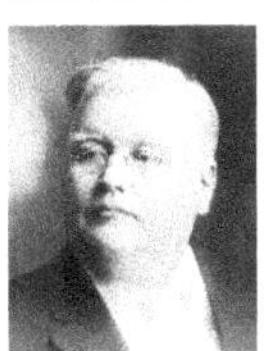

Henry Lindlahr M.D.
1862–1924
Integrated diet, sun, exercise, hydrotherapy; opened the naturopathic college

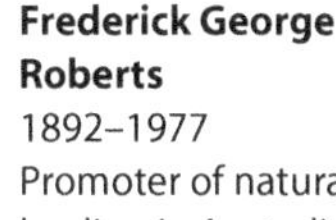

Leslie Owen Bailey
1890–1964
Founded The Natural Health Society of Australia and Hopewood House

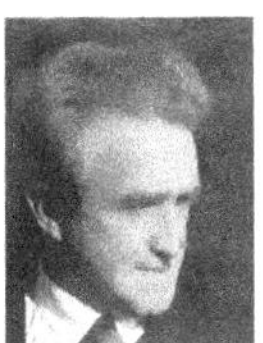

James C. Thompson
1887–1960
Co-founded Nature Cure Association; ran Kingston Clinic, Scotland

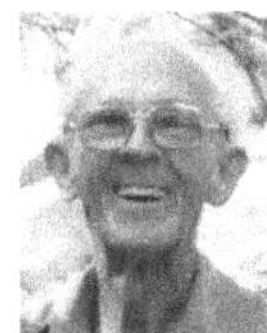

Kenneth S. Jaffrey
1909–1998
Synthesized Nature Cure teachings; lectured & published widely; trained over thirty naturopaths

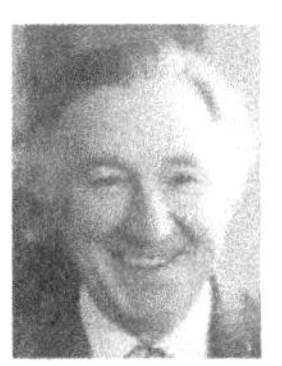

Leslie C. Thompson
1919–1992
Continued Kingston Clinic after father's death

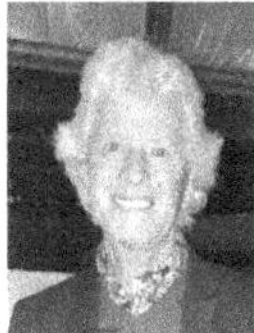

Kevin D. Hinton
1932–2017
Student of Jaffrey, teacher, and writer, who carried forward the Nature Cure philosophy and hydrotherapy practice. He trained the author among many other students.

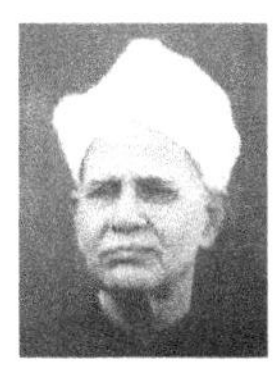

K. Lakshmana Sarma
1879–1965
Father of Nature Cure in India; promoted self-treatment including hydrotherapy

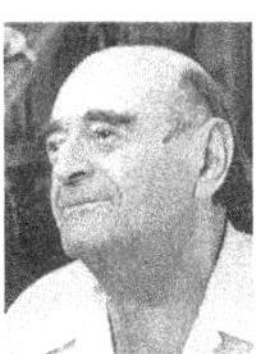

Prof. Edmond Bordeaux Székely
1905–1979
Developed Cosmotherapy, a scientific basis for naturopathy

As you will see in the next chapter, the same simple physiological principles Priessnitz intuited remain unchanged in the twenty-first century.

From this brief history we see that hydrotherapy has roots in both ancient and modern civilizations. Despite centuries of change, the central idea remains: health is restored when we cooperate with nature, not oppose it.

And so, with history as our foundation, let us now turn to the simple science behind hydrotherapy – the physiological principles that explain why these age-old practices remain so effective.

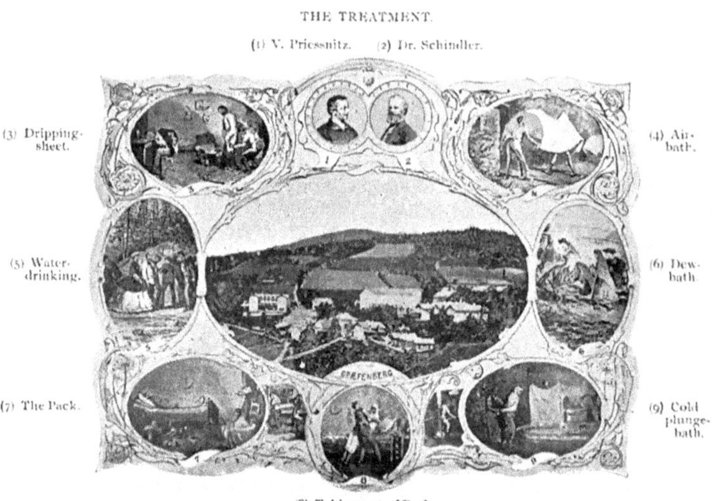

(8) Taking out of Pack.

Chapter Three

The Scientific Basis of Hydrotherapy

*"Healing is not a science, a trade or an art. Healing is
a process that occurs when conditions are favourable,
providing the injury is not excessively severe."*
Kenneth S. Jaffrey

What is the true scientific basis of hydrotherapy? What exactly happens inside the body, and on its surface, when a hydropathic treatment is applied? Answering these questions is what this chapter is all about.

I still recall my high school science lessons where we were taught certain irrefutable principles. Among them was this: all living organisms are **self-regulating, self-reproducing, and self-healing**. This simple truth applies to the tiniest cell as well as the most complex body. Physics adds another foundational principle: **heat expands and cold contracts**. This law applies universally to all matter, including human tissue.

Heat and Cold: The Physiological Pump

When cold water is applied to the body, its thermic effect causes contraction of the muscle and skin tissue. This reaction increases circulation and encourages drainage from the treated area. In contrast, heat produces expansion, relaxing tissue and drawing blood toward the surface. When these applications are alternated with heat followed by cold, they create a natural *physiological pump*, dramatically improving blood flow and lymphatic movement.

It is important to remember that **heat relaxes and sedates, while cold stimulates and invigorates**. However, extremes in either direction can be harmful. Excessive heat overstimulates and weakens tissue, while overuse of cold can oppress vitality and even cause damage. The art of hydrotherapy lies in applying these forces with balance, precision, and sensitivity to the patient's vitality.

Székely on the Triple Role of Water

The great Professor Edmond Székely you can read about in *Cosmos, Man & Society* page 493, (1936), described the effects of hydrotherapy in these words:

"As it is the nature of disease to have its origins in disturbances of the blood caused either by irregular, defective circulation, or the presence of foreign, morbific elements, our methods (hydrotherapeutic), being based on the foregoing principle, water has the triple object of:

1. Dissolving the toxic substances in the bloodstream

2. Eliminating these toxic elements from the human body

3. Strengthening and invigorating the system, and ultimately restoring regular circulation to the purified blood."

Székely's insight reinforces what Nature Cure has always taught us. That water itself has no healing power as it is merely the medium. Healing occurs when the body (if sufficiently vital and placed under the right conditions) responds to these applications. Hydrotherapy simply assists in creating and maintaining these favourable conditions.

The Role of Metabolism in Healing

The actual healing process is carried out by the body's own metabolism. Waste must be mobilised, liquefied, and excreted. Proper circulation ensures that nutrients are delivered to cells while toxins are removed. Hydrotherapy acts as an *aid* to this process, not a replacement for it.

Three Physiological Effects of Hydrotherapy

The effects of water therapy can be grouped into three categories:

1. **Thermal Effects** – produced by applying water above or below normal body temperature. The further the difference from 37°C (98.6°F), the greater the response will be, provided the individual's vitality allows their body to respond to it.

2. **Mechanical Effects** – caused by the physical force of water in forms such as sprays, douches, frictions, immersions, or compresses. These forces stimulate skin, nerves, and circulation directly.

3. **Chemical Effects** – arising when water is ingested internally or used to irrigate body cavities. This includes its solvent action in diluting and flushing out impurities.

Of these, the thermal and mechanical effects form the foundation of hydrotherapy and are the primary concern of this book.

Chronic Disease and the Need for Hydrotherapy

Whenever the free flow of blood, lymph, and nerve force is obstructed, the body falls into a state of chronic disease. This stagnation of circulation is at the root of most long-term illness. Hydrotherapy, by stimulating flow and drainage, directly addresses this obstruction.

Yet, it must be stressed: hydrotherapy is not a stand-alone cure. It is one tool among many in the Nature Cure practice. A competent practitioner will always recommend broader lifestyle corrections in the way of removing causes of disease, restoring natural habits, and supporting vitality, while using hydrotherapy to assist the return to normality.

With this scientific foundation in mind, we can now explore the various practical applications of hydrotherapy from simple home treatments to the more advanced techniques historically developed in Nature Cure clinics. These methods, when applied with intelligence and consistency, serve as powerful aids in restoring the body's natural balance.

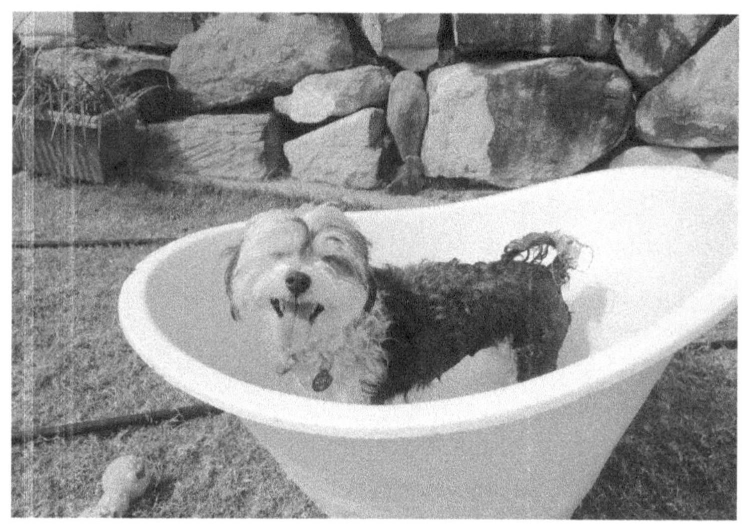

Hip or Dog Bath

Applications of Hydrotherapy

"Water is life's matter and matrix, mother and medium.
There is no life without water"
Albert Szent-Györgyi

I have found that hydrotherapy is both a science and an art that should be learned by each individual to suit their own specific health needs. To that end, hydrotherapy treatments (among other lifestyle adjustments) should be recommended by a competent Nature Cure practitioner or Hydrotherapist.

Fundamentally, hydrotherapy is simply the use of water to achieve cleanliness, muscle tone and balance (an equalising if you will), of bodily fluids and nerve force. Water should be used in a non-invasive way by employing baths and compresses. The safest and most valuable treatments are vapour baths, hip/sitz baths, spinal baths, cold compresses and packs. These water treatments can assist greatly in the relief of pain and in achieving and maintaining health when they are correctly applied.

There are times when hydropathic treatments **should not** be used. They are:

1. If the patient has a weakened heart condition

2. If the patient is frail and unable to garner a reaction

3. If the patient has high blood pressure

4. If the patient is unable to adjust to cool or high temperatures

5. If the patient is suffering from an acute illness involving fever.

As with any therapeutic treatment, there are guidelines that should be adhered to for the best results to be achieved, these include:

1. Never apply an extreme temperature (hot or cold) to the skin/body.

2. Every action of water on the body must be followed by an equal and opposite reaction through a variation in temperature. For example, if using heat, finish with cold, or vice versa.

3. Cold water application must never be applied while the person already feels chilled. Cold water is invigorating only if we possess the vitality to provoke the desired reaction.

4. When possible, take a moment to dry skin brush all parts of the body before any application as this will provide the best opportunity for the skin to eliminate waste matter. NB: The skin is the largest organ of elimination.

5. Never use water applications within one hour before or after a meal.

6. Only drink water when thirsty (most of the water required by the body is contained within a standard natural diet of fruits and vegetables).

7. If subject to great tension and stress and muscles are spastic, drink warm water.

8. Cold baths should always be taken alternately with a sun bath or warming treatment.

9. Marathon baths are used to detoxify the body. These are showers of hot water that pass over the whole body for long periods. These baths are enervating and should only be used in emergencies in order to detoxify the body quickly, such as in the case of acute poisoning. Steam baths have the same effect but are much less enervating.

The bottom line is that there are various treatments in the hydrotherapy tool kit, and they all have their own specific applications. Yet, their purpose is the same. All treatments of hydrotherapy assist in providing unimpeded circulation of blood, lymph and nerve force. After a comprehensive diagnosis from your Nature Cure practitioner, you will likely receive recommendations for one or more of the following hydropathic treatments:

1. Local compresses
2. A full body wrap/compress
3. Steam/vapour baths
4. Clay packs
5. Foot Bath
6. Hip/sitz bath
7. Spinal baths
8. Piecemeal baths.

A General Guide to the use of Compresses

I'm going to cover some general points first. Best results are achieved when applications are performed consistently and in accordance with directions from your Nature Cure practitioner. Where possible, you should learn to apply all compresses by yourself (age permitting). If required, it is best to have a friend or someone nearby nursing you.

The two main pieces of material required for compresses include:

1. Cotton material which acts as the conductor, which means that it creates a reaction with the skin. An old sheet can be cut to the desired size required for each treatment.

2. Woollen material which acts as an insulator (it insulates the cotton material to maintain the cool reaction for as long as possible with the skin). Old woollen blankets can be cut to size for each treatment.

Other items that are useful are ice gel bags, clay packs, hot water bottles, electric heat pads and quality natural fibre socks.

Tips for compressing:

- The length of time to wear a compress varies. Usually, two hours or when the cotton material dries out and becomes uncomfortable to wear are the signs that indicate it's time to finish.
- Place the wet cotton material in the fridge to cool the material down further for those in warmer climates. This will induce the desired reaction.
- The compress is a beneficial treatment for those suffering from poor circulation in the affected area, and/or those who have suffered an injury or trauma of some kind.
- Whenever a local compress is used, a complimentary waist compress should be applied.
- Consistency of application is the rule for all compressing if you wish to achieve the best results.
- For convenience, you could apply the compress while you are reading a book, using an electronic device or watching television.
- Having a warm shower prior to wearing a compress will provide the desired reaction without causing a chill to the skin.
- It is always best to rest while wearing any compress for optimum effectiveness to expedite the repair of an injury. The value-add here is that it benefits the whole body, not just the injured area.

The more energy conserved during the healing process via *The Principle of The Conservation of Energy*, the speedier the recovery will be. It's important to note that we are not just treating the injured area in the practice of hydrotherapy. We are treating the body as a whole. Here the *Principle of Unity* applies when we are encouraging the healing process.

The Different Types of Compresses

There are a number of different applications when using compresses to aid healing and recovery. We're going to take a look at the main approaches here.

Local Compresses

Compresses may be applied to any part of the body. These are called local compresses. Whenever a local compress is applied to a specific part of the body, it is best to apply a complimentary compress around the waist in the location of the kidneys. This will draw the waste matter to this area and assist in its elimination.

Foot/Feet Compress

Materials include the following:

- Cotton socks
- Minimum of three woollen booties.

How to apply: Wet the cotton sock/s and wring them out as much as possible. Once you have the cotton socks on your foot/feet, quickly put on a minimum of three layers of woollen socks/booties. Lie down immediately and rest.

Leg Compress

This compress can cover different parts of the leg, including the thigh, knee, lower leg and ankles.

Materials include the following:

- Cotton material to wrap around the area, once only

- Woollen material that will wrap around the area at least three times.

How to apply: Wet enough cotton material to enable the compress to cover an area six times the size of the affected area being treated. Then wring out the excess water and place the compress in the fridge to cool down further if required. Wrap one layer of the cotton material around the leg and wrap the woollen material around the area being treated three to four times and fasten it with a safety pin or Velcro.

Waist Compress or Complimentary Compress
Materials include the following:

- Cotton cloth 30cm wide in a length that is sufficient to wrap around the area being treated once only
- Woollen material 4m in length folded over a number of times to result in eight layers of wool.

How to apply: Soak the cotton cloth in cold water. Wring it out well and wrap one layer around the waist. Wrap the woollen material over the cotton cloth, providing at least four layers of coverage, and fix it with a pin or Velcro.

Hand Compress
Required materials:

- A long cotton sock or cotton glove
- Woollen Gloves or wool material approximately 2m long, double layered to achieve four layers of wool.

How to apply: Soak the cotton material in cold water. Wring it out well and slip your hand into the sock or glove, or wrap it in the woollen material several times, then fix it to hold the compress in place.

Neck Compress

Required materials:

- Cotton cloth 4cm wide x approximately 30cm long
- Woollen material that is wider than the cotton cloth and long enough to wrap around the neck three to four times.

How to apply: Soak the cotton cloth in cold water. Wring it out well and wrap it around the neck. Then wrap the woollen material over the cotton cloth, around the neck several times and fix it with a pin or Velcro to secure it.

Eye Compress

Materials required:

- Cotton cloth 4cm x 30cm
- Woollen material is wider than the cotton cloth and long enough to wrap around the eyes/head three to four times.

How to apply: Soak the cotton cloth in cold water. Wring it out well and wrap it around the eyes. Then wrap the woollen material over the cotton cloth, and wrap it around the eyes three times before fixing it with a pin or Velcro to secure it.

Full Body Wrap/Compress

The full body wrap usually follows a full body heat treatment, like a hot shower or preferably a steam bath. We then follow the heat treatment with a cool application to maximize the benefit. Options include a cool shower, a plunge bath or the full body compress. The latter has been proven to produce the best results.

When it comes to the full body wrap/compress, you will need one double bed size cotton sheet, four to six pure woollen blankets, and an area wide enough for a person to lay down on comfortably. The floor or a bed usually works best.

To set up for the full body wrap, lay the blankets one on top of the other on the treatment table or floor, so that you'll have a stack of blankets under you or the person you are treating. Then wet the cotton sheet and wring all of the excess water out of it (you can do this on a slow, short spin cycle in your washing machine), then lay the damp sheet on top of the blankets.

On completion of the steam bath, immediately have the patient lie down on their back on the pile of blankets topped with the damp sheet. Tuck the damp sheet around the patient from their neck to their feet, ensuring it makes contact with all areas of their skin. Then wrap the woollen blankets over the patient.

Encourage the patient to relax and breathe rhythmically and diaphragmatically. The time taken for this treatment is generally around 30 minutes for most people. However, it can go for longer if they wish, until the sheet is dry, which is usually about 60 minutes.

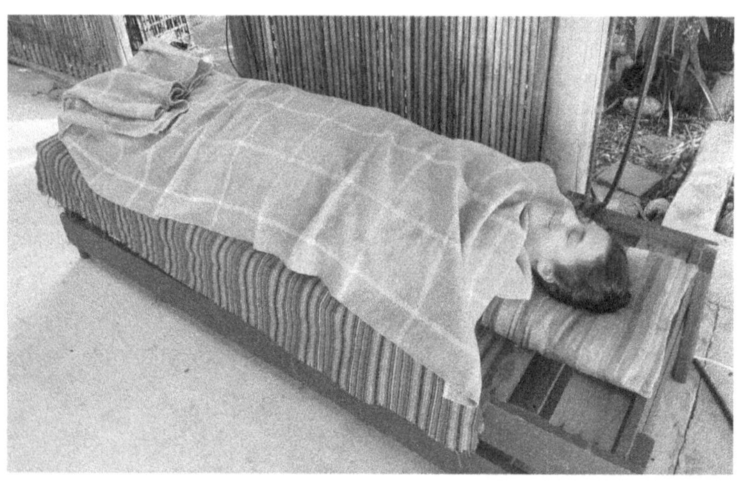

Patient wrapped up in a full body compress

When the time is up, remove the patient from the body wrap, have them shower before laying down for a short rest. This completes this treatment.

Then it's time to wash the sheet and hang the blankets out to dry in the sunshine while you clean out the steam bath.

Clay Pack

A clay pack is similar to the cold compress, except clay holds moisture for longer than a cotton compress. It is most useful for treating symptoms deep in the body, for example, bones or tumours. It has naturally absorbent properties that aid in the healing process. It will act faster and with deeper penetration than a regular cloth compress. The time factor for healing will be accelerated greatly by the use of a clay pack.

How to apply: Mix a portion of clay with water until it is a sticky consistency similar to dough. Put a cricket ball size piece of this clay onto the affected body part. Spread it with a utensil keeping your hands clean. Cover it with a piece of moist cotton cloth, then cover that with several layers of woollen material. Change the clay pack when it has dried out.

When to apply: The best time to apply a clay pack is before retiring. You will find that it has dried out upon waking. The clay pack is also very good for dealing with things like snakebites, or in the case of being injected with the venom of marine stingers, wasps, bees or hornets. The clay will draw out poisons from the bites much faster and more efficiently than a regular compress does.

NOTE: The clay does not deteriorate and can be reused time and time again. Simply break up the dry clay and mix it with cold water, and it will be ready for you to apply it again. Kaolin clay can generally be purchased from chemists or online.

The Different Types of Baths

Steam or Vapor Baths

It's best to seek the recommendation of a qualified Nature Cure practitioner or Hydrotherapist when embarking on your first experience of a Steam Bath. It is an enclosed structure with a heating element and water to create steam in order to open the pores of the skin and increase the circulation. It is used by those who wish to remove impurities from their skin and to relax their nervous system. Various disease conditions will benefit from the use of a steam bath.

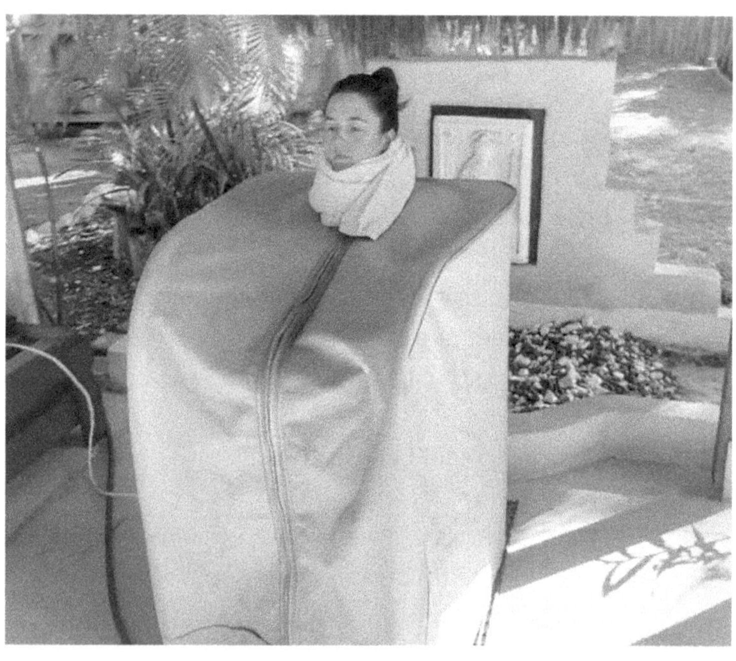

Laura (my daughter) in portable canvas steam bath

How to take a steam bath

Fill the bath with water to the marked level on the container, and preheat the steam unit before getting in. Cover the opening with a towel to contain the steam being generated. While this is happening, give your body an all over dry skin brush. This will remove dead skin cells, stimulate blood flow to the surface of the skin, and open up the pores in your skin in preparation for the steam bath. It is recommended that no clothing is worn, and that you have a towel to sit on and a towel to wrap around your neck in order to contain the steam within the bath chamber.

As far as the length of time in the steam bath goes, it's best to remove the patient (or yourself) when the temporal pressure increases, or alternatively when perspiration appears on their upper lip. Obviously if the patient is feeling overheated, claustrophobic or uncomfortable in some other way, it's time to bring the session to an end.

*It is recommended to have an assistant present at all times during this treatment.

Foot Bath

The purpose of a foot bath is to increase circulation and enable drainage with the aim of relieving pain and discomfort in the feet in particular, and relaxing the nervous system in general. For example, headaches are a result of pressure in the temporal area due to excess blood and poor circulation, therefore standing in a bath of cold water, walking on wet grass, walking in a cool stream or the ocean, will relieve the pressure by increasing blood flow to the opposite end of the body, away from the temporal area.

The foot bath also assists certain conditions such as arthritis and related skin diseases on the feet. Ultimately, as with all hydrotherapy applications, the aim is to assist in the removal of obstructions to the free flow of blood lymph and nerve force to the areas in question. In terms of the best time to take a foot bath, the answer is that anytime of the day is suitable. Personally, I have found that the best time to take this bath is just before retiring. I'm not alone in this preference though, because quite simply, it's a most soothing tonic for a restful sleep.

How to take a foot bath: Take two small tubs/buckets which will hold enough water for your feet to sit flat and the water level to reach the ankles. Fill one of the tubs with cold water and the other one with hot water (at a temperature that will not scald the skin). Starting with the hot water, rest both feet in the bath for three minutes. Then place your feet into the cold bath for one minute. Repeat this for at least three cycles which will equate to a total treatment time of 15 minutes or longer if desired. Upon completion, dry your feet and prepare to retire for the day, or rest for a period of no less than 30 minutes if possible.

A complementary treatment that can be added after the foot bath involves applying foot compresses and wearing them to bed (refer to feet compress section for more information about this). Empty the baths, clean them out, and store them for next time.

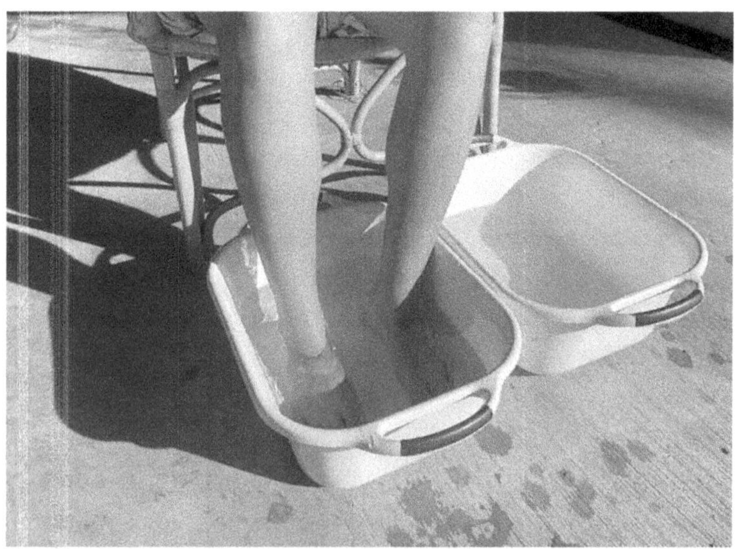

Sitz/Hip Bath

The sitz bath, which is otherwise known as the hip bath, has its origins back in 1842. The word 'sitz' is derived from the German word *Sitzbad*, meaning a bath *(bad)* in which one sits *(sitzen)*. Such hip baths were originally a European custom. The bath itself is a receptacle that holds water deep enough to sit in with the water reaching the navel and top half of the legs.

Note: an alternative to the bath is to use a large plastic storage container that accommodates your size.

The purpose of the hip bath is to increase blood circulation to the digestive and reproductive areas. It is also used by those who are wishing to calm their nervous system and lower their body heat on a hot day.

When to take a Hip Bath: The best time of day to take a hip bath is in the morning sun, usually before 10 am and well before the midday sun, to coincide with the circadian cycle of elimination and excretion within the human body.

How to take a cool water hip bath: Start by ensuring the patient (or yourself as the case may be) is sufficiently warm. This is an opportune time to take in the solar radiations, warming up the body before the cooling bath. Or you could take a walk and increase your circulation to tap into the best reactions. Then, when you are ready, sit in the bath, facing the early morning sun or late afternoon sun.

You can take the treatment outdoors or indoors. Fill the bath two-thirds of the way to the top with cool tap water. If you live in a warm climate where your tap water is only lukewarm, it is advisable to put ice or ice packs in the bath to cool the water down. Remember the whole aim of hydrotherapy is to induce a reaction in the body. Once seated in the bath, the water level should reach up to the navel (this will depend on the amount of water your body displaces once you are seated). It is best to wear minimal clothing, especially if you are partaking in the morning sun at the same time.

Wearing a hat is advisable when outdoors. Conversely, if you are in an environment with cold ambient weather, you can wear a thick jumper on your top half, slippers on your feet, and put a blanket over your legs. I say that because we only want to induce cool into the area of the body immersed in the bath.

The duration of the bath will be determined by the reaction of the individual to the cool water. I suggest you start with a period of 5 – 10 minutes. Adjust the time as you progress. Then remove yourself from the hip bath and dry the wet area and observe the length of time it takes for the chilled area to warm back up. Lay down, stay warm and rest if you're tired.

I can't think of a more productive and beneficial way to start the day.

Much can be accomplished that revolves around this treatment. When taking an omnilateral (many sided) approach, this treatment can be used with other health building elements, including deep rhythmic breathing. This is likely to bring about mental poise while you're bathing in the sunlight, feet on the wet grass taking in the benefits of the treatment itself.

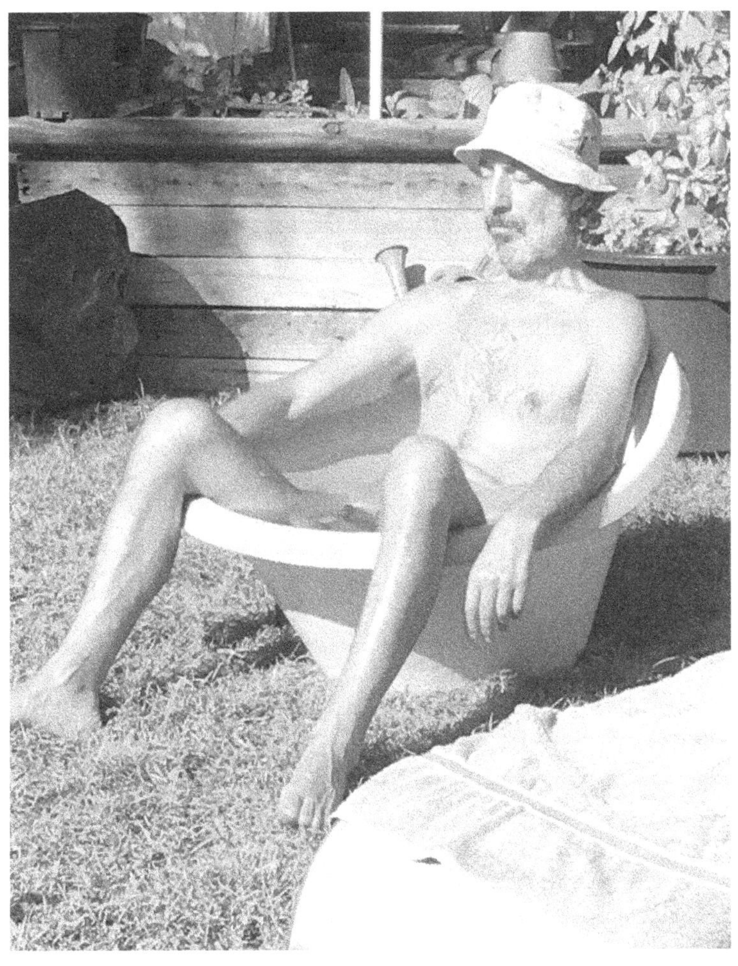

Morning Hip Bath

Spinal Bath and Combined Use of the Elements

The history of the modern spinal bath design originated with K. Lakshmana Sarma who is known as the Father of Nature Cure in India. He is a man who contributed greatly to the Nature Cure movement worldwide. His most remarkable invention was the spinal bathtub that was made out of metal. The design was taken by Mr Kenneth Jaffrey and subsequently modified by my teacher Kevin Hinton. These tubs are now being made from a lightweight fibreglass material with a far more comfortable design, allowing for a degree of neck depression as shown in the images below. This image shows the wet cotton towel positioned along the spine and rolled at the neck for comfort.

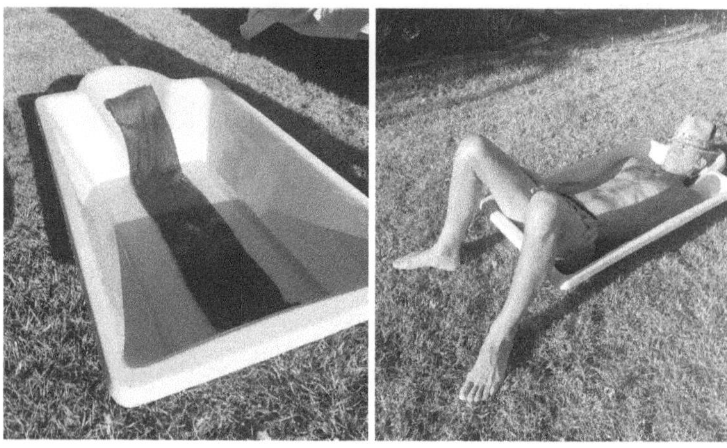

Afternoon spinal bath…the best treatment for the spine and nervous system from years of experience!

As far as definitions go, a spinal bath is ideally a receptacle or a wet towel that is long enough and wide enough to touch the spine from the neck to the tailbone with **cool** water.

What is the purpose of the spinal bath? Quite simply, its purpose is to assist with circulation through the spinal column to aid in relaxing the nervous system. It is beneficial for certain conditions such as enervation, restlessness or agitation, depression, spinal subluxations and disc injuries. This treatment is best applied with minimal clothing so as not to impede the intended circulatory direction.

When is the best time to perform this treatment? Either early morning or in the late afternoon tends to work best. I have found after three is a suitable time in the subtropics, or at other times indoors to suit your circumstances.

Ensure you are warm in preparation for the bath. I suggest taking a sunbath to the back, or a walk, or a warm shower with the water focused on the spine, to increase your circulation, then as you ease yourself into the cool bath, you should feel the need for an initial gasp of air as your skin reacts to the cold water. Start with 5-10 minutes and adjust the time you spend as you progress, allowing as much time as you feel comfortable. You should be paying attention to how you are feeling throughout the process. Are you starting to feel a chill? If so then it's time to get out. You are always looking for the reaction, or as Kevin would often say, "listen to the voice of the organism", and let this be your guide.

It was Professor Székely who coined the term *Cosmovital Bath*, which included the elements of sun, air and water. The knowledge to combine these elements was discovered by Székely during an archaeological dig of Sumerian grave sites where he found the Sumerian baths. These were formed in the shape of the body dug into the clay ground and filled with water.

To emulate the Sumerian bath, if your environment allows for it, I would suggest an omnilateral approach to the spinal bath treatment described above. This will elevate your experience and afford the most beneficial results over time.

The first element of this practice involves you lying face down on the grass with your feet pointing towards the sun, absorbing the subtle **terrestrial radiations**. You'll rest here for a while exposing your back, as you take in the second element of essential **solar radiations**.

Once you've set everything up and you are ready to start, lay down in the spinal bath with your feet facing the sun. As you rest and relax, breathe in the third element as you inhale deep breaths of **air**. Without needing to do anything extra, you will be taking in the fourth element in the form of **water** while you're lying down in the spinal bath of cool water that's approximately 5 cm in depth with the folded cotton towel running along the full length of your spine, tucked through your legs to the genitals and a small roll at the neck to support the cervical curvature ensuring comfort.

In this one treatment, these elements of earth, sun, air, and water combine to engage the fifth element in the form of **mental poise**. When practicing this treatment, it's a good opportunity to begin a deep rhythmic breathing cycle, as you relax and develop your vision of a happy nurturing place. I'd urge you to allow as much time as you can for this treatment, as you may drift off into the calm state of rest that will rejuvenate your nervous system. This is a most powerful regenerative process.

When you have completed the treatment, have a dry towel ready to briskly rub up and down the length of the spine. Allow some time to lie down on your stomach exposing your back to the sun again, warming the area that has been cooled whilst in the spinal bath (see image below).

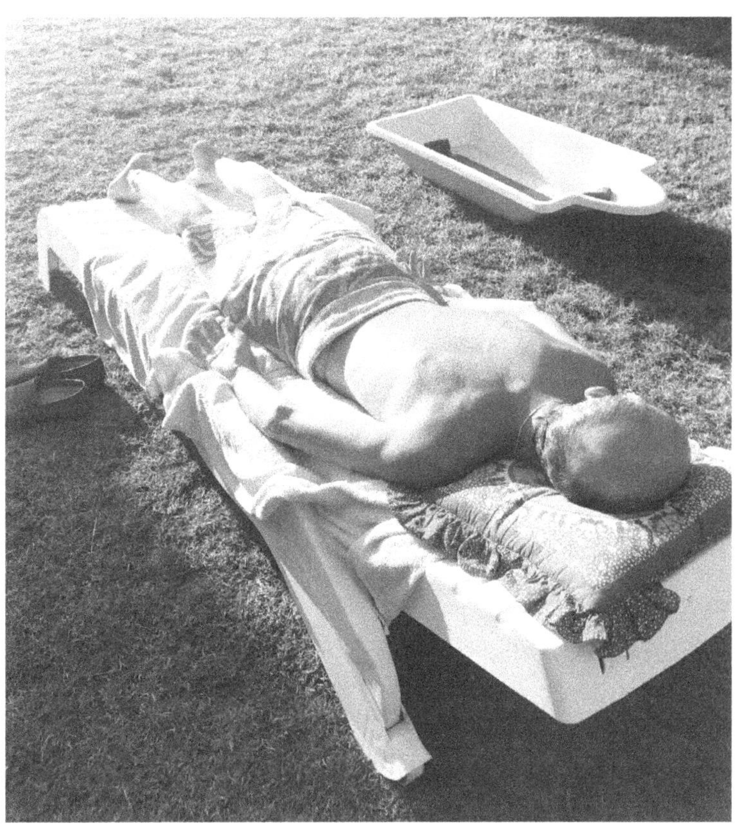

The period immediately after a spinal bath is a time to rest, relax and stay warm while slowing the chatter of the mind as you become acutely aware of the sounds of nature. This is a great environment to focus on your breath and allow yourself to become fully present.

An alternative to using a spinal bath is to place a dry towel down on the ground and then position a long folded wet towel (which has been rung out) onto the dry towel and lie down with your spine in contact with the wet towel – just as I described when using the folded towel in the spinal bath. You could use a sunlounge in a similar way. This treatment can be done inside if the weather is not suitable to do it outside.

Avoid chilling yourself at all costs by covering yourself with a blanket and using heat packs on your feet. I say that because we only want the spine cooled during a spinal bath.

If you regularly take advantage of spinal baths, you will find that over a period of time your circulation, skin tone and texture, wellbeing and mental poise will show marked improvements. More broadly, if you maintain a natural lifestyle, your health will continue to improve and you will come to experience the added bonus of having an inner smile that develops as a result of feeling well!

Now think about what this will cost you. In anyone's language it is great value. I say that because pretty much it is only your time and effort that you need to invest to get some truly amazing results. That's an excellent return on investment, don't you think?

Piecemeal Bath

Also known as a friction bath, the piecemeal Bath is a simple treatment that can be done in any situation. It is considered a general application. The purpose of the piecemeal bath is to stimulate circulation to all parts of the body. It involves taking a basin of cold water and putting your hands in it, then rubbing the part of the body to be treated. Begin with the hands and move from the top of the body downward over the entire body, one section at a time, rubbing each part of the body until your wet hands become dry.

This treatment benefits those who have skin problems such as psoriasis, dermatitis, eczema or poor skin more generally. It is also beneficial for those who are enervated and of a nervous disposition. After completion of this treatment rub the whole body down vigorously with a dry towel and take some time to rest.

First Aid – Hydrotherapy for Treating Physical Injuries

My eldest son was a professional dancer, and my daughter was a semi-professional soccer player. They have occasionally had injuries in the way of bumps and bruises to their knee, ankle, neck, head etc., and have used compresses to expedite their recovery. They have both acknowledged the efficacy of this treatment from their personal experiences with hydrotherapy and continue to apply this in their everyday lives.

It's not uncommon to hear about the use of ice on bruises for all manner of trauma. Have you ever stopped to think about what is actually happening to create the results you achieve when you use ice? What happens is that ice cold treatments numb the fine capillaries, muscle tissue and nerves … aarrrhh the nerves. So essentially, we are deadening the pain so that we can get back on the footy field, dance floor, workplace, etc.

It's important to note that using ice on an injury can cause harm to the tissue and nerves in the long term. This is because ice constricts the blood vessels, deadens the nerves and reduces the blood flow to the injured area, and in so doing, it impedes the healing process. On the other hand, a compress, foot bath or any suitable hydrotherapy application does not have the kinds of instant results applying ice to an injury might have, but it is a gentler and a less harmful way of reducing pain and swelling.

The capacity for cells to renew fully is not up for dispute. And we know that humans are not designed to survive in extremes of either cold or heat. So, it's important to note that there's a cost relating to the fact that our pain is being diminished because our nerves are being deadened by the ice. When this happens, we are stressing our body in a way that a natural gentler option of taking a warm shower and lying down simply does not do.

For example, if it's a foot injury you're dealing with, you'll be doing yourself a favour by applying a compress to the injured area and raising that foot on a pillow. This approach assists in increasing the blood flow to the affected area and allowing the healing process to take place. The application of heat packs for three minutes, followed by a cold pack for one minute is an alternative to a compress. The longer you are able to rest, the greater and sooner the reduction to the pain you will experience. I'd suggest you lie down for at least 24 hours consuming as little as possible or preferably just sipping pure water. The body will heal best when minimal exertion is practised.

You'll need to change the compress every 2–3 hours, and the swelling and pain will slowly diminish without any of the trauma that the use of ice is likely to promote.

Using a hot water bottle, heated wheat pack or heat pad placed at your feet in bed in the evenings will provide the nerve endings at the bottom of your feet with a soothing tonic for a good night's rest. Re-educate yourself to a gentler way of restoring your body.

Hygiene Tips:
I've included some points below to assist maintaining a hygienic practices of hydrotherapy.

- Use your own intelligence in determining water temperature as the objective is not to chill the body.
- On the completion of a compress treatment, hang the woollen material out to air in the sun and wash the cotton material.
- After a steam bath, wipe down the steam cabinet and leave it open to air out. Hang out all woollen blankets in the sun preferably, and wash the cotton sheet.
- After the use of the hip bath or spinal bath, empty the water and allow it to dry. With the spinal bath, wring out the towel and hang it out to dry for the next use.

In Kevin and Katy Hinton's book titled *A Lifestyle for Health & Happiness*, there are seven pages dedicated to hydrotherapy that provide a very effective short overview. I highly recommend reading not just this section of the book but the whole book, which gives a complete understanding of a natural lifestyle. (See the References on page 67 at the end of this book to access a copy.)

For further reading on the various uses for compresses and hydrotherapy, I encourage you to read *Naturopathic First Aid* by Kenneth S. Jaffrey. The text below that I am quoting to sign off on this chapter is by Eric Karlsson ND DN who was a student of Jaffrey, based in Sweden with patients from around Europe.

"In hydrotherapy, water is used in different ways; for example, steam baths, sitz baths, spinal baths, cold body packs and local compresses. The purpose is to dissolve and assist in the elimination of poisonous substances (toxins), stored in the body tissue through increasing blood circulation. Hydrotherapy can be used in many ways. Hydrotherapy must be used correctly and very individually. When done so, it is often very effective."

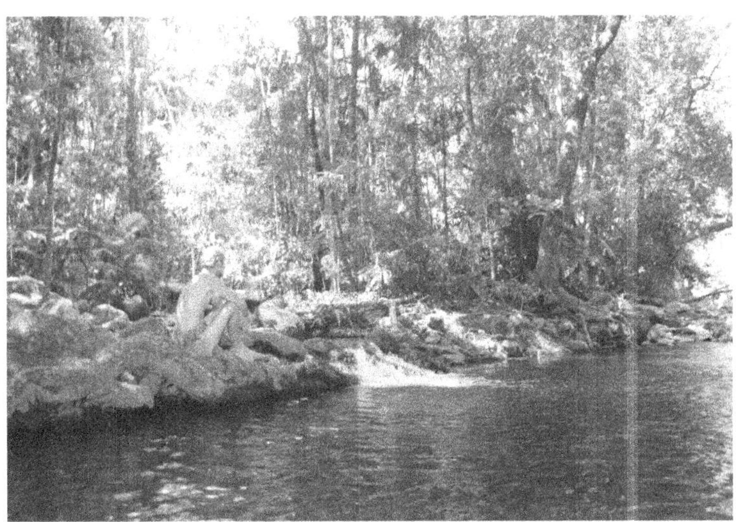

Chapter Five

True Story – Healing Through Hydrotherapy

To Debra, who survived the crash with me – may your recovery be full and complete, in every way.

Just as I was preparing to send this manuscript to my publisher for editing and publication, life took a sudden turn. I was involved in a serious motor vehicle crash. From this collision I was left with a severe concussion and numerous broken bones, including my ankle, collarbone, ribs, sternum, and fractures to several vertebrae.

There's no need to go into all the details, but while I was in hospital getting through the critical stages of recovery, I often recalled the injuries suffered by Priessnitz back in the 1820s. How he approached his recovery was no different to the way I chose to approach mine, except I had the benefit of the added knowledge passed down from our forefathers, making it more accessible and practical for us to use today.

What follows are the very treatments I applied to myself, which greatly supported and accelerated my healing journey.

From the earliest days in hospital, I used the hand-held shower rose with alternating hot and cold applications on my shoulder, back, neck, and chest. Each session always ended with cold water applied for as long as I could tolerate it, usually no longer than a minute. This was followed by a brisk rubdown and a return to bed with freshly prepared sheets, a small but meaningful comfort. Sitting by the window for a change of view became a daily delight. I often recalled the words of Dr. Hilton: *"Pain is the monitor; rest is the cure."* In these circumstances, his wisdom rang profoundly true, as I found that all I wanted to do was just rest.

After a few weeks, I was transferred to a smaller regional hospital. There, the grounds offered a more restorative environment with fresh air, fruit trees, tropical flowers alive with butterflies and birds. It was a sanctuary of nature's beauty, and blessedly quieter than the city. Rest in hospital is rarely easy, so I learned to sleep whenever my body permitted it. Many mornings were spent reclining in the sunlit gardens, with my wounds exposed to the healing rays of the sun. Once the wounds healed and bandages were removed from my leg, the hot-and-cold shower routine was extended to my ankle as well.

Upon returning home, I developed a daily regimen that included neck, waist, and leg compresses applied while resting, reading, or watching a program. I also used a gentle slant board in the morning and afternoon to relieve pressure on my spine and promote circulation between my vertebrae. Hot and cold foot baths became invaluable, both for stimulating blood flow and easing pain in my injured ankle, as well as encouraging rapid healing of scar tissue.

One of the simplest yet most effective tools was the humble hot water bottle. With the head trauma and spinal injuries affecting my nervous system – the very system that links all others – the nightly application of the hot water bottle to my feet proved invaluable. A warm thank you to the nurses who assisted with this application while in hospital. The warmth soothed the thousands of nerve endings and promoted deep relaxation and rest. The shower also continued to play an important role in stimulating circulation, particularly for my fractured cervical vertebrae. Once warmed by the water, I could gently rotate my neck, encouraging movement and reduced pain.

When I was finally strong enough, I added spinal baths to my afternoon routine, often after enjoying a long sunbath.

Throughout this period, hydrotherapy was not my only source

of support. I also worked closely with physiotherapists performing relevant stretches and exercises, as well as chiropractors for the gentle re alignment of the vertebrae, along with surgeons and other specialists. Yet, I am convinced that hydrotherapy significantly accelerated my recovery, greatly reducing pain and restoring mobility far sooner than expected by my treating physicians. The recovery is ongoing.

I remain deeply grateful for the timeless knowledge handed down through our natural healing traditions. It continues to sustain me during one of the greatest trials of my life, and it is now my hope that this story inspires you to explore these simple yet powerful methods. Use them, trust them, and reap their benefits for your own health and vitality.

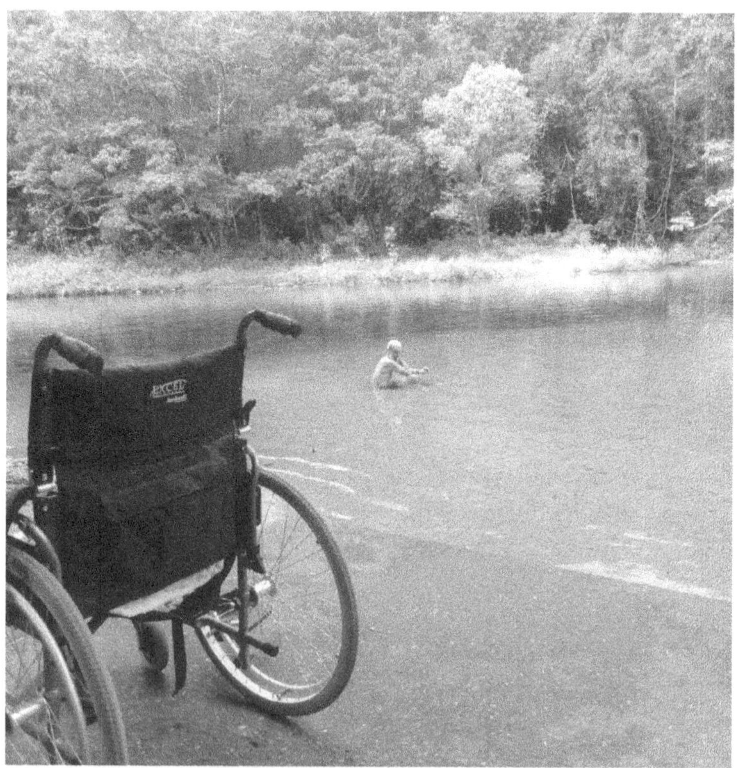

Chapter Six

Hydrotherapy in Nature Cure

*"Nothing is softer or more flexible than
water, yet nothing can resist it."*
Lao Tzu

This chapter explains where hydrotherapy fits into the larger story of Natural Living and Natural Healing that is often referred to as *Nature Cure*. As we touched on in Chapter Three, hydrotherapy, or as it was popularly called in the 1800s, *The Water Cure*, laid the foundation for what has since evolved into Nature Cure. Importantly, the teachings of Nature Cure – whether you call them Pure Naturopathy, Natural Hygiene, Hydrotherapy, or simply The Water Cure are not the fleeting notions of one individual. Rather, they are the distilled wisdom of generations who observed the laws of life and health at work.

My teacher, Kevin D. Hinton, often reminded his students that *"The health of a human being is determined by two factors. One is our hereditary disposition, and the other is the environment in which we live."*

Of course, none of us can alter our genetic inheritance, but we can influence, to a very great degree, the environment and lifestyle we choose to live in. The point I want to stress here is that our environment is not limited to things like geography or climate. It is the sum total of every physical and mental influence surrounding us. These influences reach us through the senses, shaping our state of health. What this means is that by consciously choosing to live healthfully, we do not just improve our own well-being; we also provide the best foundation of health for future generations.

The Eight Essential Elements of Health

There are eight principal elements to abide by if you are seeking optimum health. Together, they form the basis of Natural Living, and hydrotherapy is one important branch of this greater tree. In brief these include:

1. Sun

The sun is the original and primary source of all life on Earth. Without its energy, no living organism could survive. Sensible exposure to sunlight – particularly in the morning and late afternoon – nourishes and strengthens the body. As children of the sun, we benefit deeply from its warmth and light. *Heliotherapy* is the word used for the treatment of disease by means of sunlight.

2. Fresh Air

The quality of the air we breathe, and the manner in which we breathe it, determine the purity and richness of our blood. A richly oxygenated bloodstream feeds every cell of the body. Fresh, clean air is a daily necessity, and learning to breathe deeply and rhythmically enhances this natural gift. *Aerotherapy* is the word used for the treatment of disease by means of breathing with intent.

3. Water

Water is the elixir of life. Every living creature depends on it, and this book is in many ways a testament to its power, both as a daily necessity and as a therapeutic tool. *Hydrotherapy*, or the application of water in its various forms, is a vital pillar of health.

4. Living Foods

Live and living foods provide nutrition and raw materials needed by the trillions of cells in the human body. It involves *what we eat, when we eat, and how we eat.* Living foods – taking in those foods closest to their natural state.

5. Exercise

Movement is essential to life. Whether it's walking, swimming, gardening, or running, exercise maintains the mobility of the body and supports its electrical and circulatory functions. Exercise performed with rhythmic breathing yields the best results. Also exercise in water has unique benefits, as buoyancy reduces gravitational strain and allows for freer movement. Just as important as activity, however, is rest after exercise.

6. Rest and Relaxation

As discussed in earlier chapters, rest is a cornerstone of healing. This is governed by the *Law of Conservation of Energy*. The most complete form of rest is sleep, when muscles release tension and energy is renewed. Yet rest extends beyond sleep. It includes periods of digestive rest, as well as daily intervals of mental quiet. During my corporate life, I often found great refreshment in placing my palms over my eyes, elbows resting on the desk, and breathing rhythmically in total darkness for five minutes. This simple practice restored clarity and vitality, allowing me to continue the day with renewed focus.

7. Mental Poise

A positive state of mind strengthens the body. While the mind does not directly control matter, it influences bodily functions and responses. A healthy body tends to produce a healthy, optimistic outlook, which in turn feeds back into the body's vitality. Mental poise – the balance of thought and feeling – is therefore an essential element of health.

8. Spinal Care

The spine is often called the 'tail of the brain'. Proper alignment of the thirty-three vertebrae ensures that nerve force flows unimpeded to every part of the body. Few things affect well-being more detrimentally than chronic back pain, which undermines both the body and spirit. Maintaining spinal integrity is indispensable for overall health.

The Muscle Car Analogy

In today's world of quick fixes, many expect overnight recovery. But this expectation is unrealistic. To illustrate this point, my teacher once compared the human body to a finely tuned muscle car with a V8 engine with eight pistons, each representing one of the natural requirements for health: sun, air, water, living foods, exercise, rest, mental poise, and spinal integrity.

So, if you treat the vehicle in the form of your body with care via the application of the equivalent of premium fuel, quality oils, regular servicing, correct tyre pressure, and sensible handling, then it will reward you with years of dependable service. On the other hand, if you neglect it by using cheap fuel, poor maintenance, and driving recklessly, problems will inevitably develop, until eventually the car breaks down altogether.

Your body is no different to a car in terms of the importance of maintenance. Nourish it according to natural laws, and it will serve you reliably for a lifetime. Abuse it, and disease is inevitable.

Neglecting any one of the eight elements is like running a V8 engine on six or seven cylinders. It may continue to function, but it will not perform at its best.

For those wishing to study these principles further, I highly recommend the book *A Lifestyle for Health and Happiness* by Kevin and Katy Hinton, available at www.naturecuresociety.org. It expands upon these eight elements in detail, providing practical guidance for living a life aligned with Nature.

Reflections

I think back to the mid-1980s, when I was a patient of Kevin and Katy Hinton at their practice in Townsville. On several occasions, I would book in for a vapour or steam bath, followed by a full-body compress. Each session lasted close to ninety minutes, leaving me deeply restored. After these treatments, I often found myself curious and wondered where this knowledge came from, and what the history behind these methods was.

While most of us have some familiarity with the steam sauna, what I experienced there was something entirely different. Kevin would always take the time to explain, opening a door into the deeper wisdom of hydrotherapy and its roots.

For most of my life, I worked in the corporate world, where I witnessed firsthand – and at times became a casualty of – the legacy of a flawed system. It is a system that demands much yet gives little to our wellbeing in return. It reminds me of a dog chasing its tail: a great deal of energy expended, but no real gain. The emphasis lies heavily on economics and productivity, often with little regard for the true health of the individual. The goal is to restore a person just enough to return them to the workforce. It's a short-term fix for a long-term problem. Frankly, it never made sense to me, and it still doesn't. It isn't even a good business model when you really think about it.

So, what is the alternative? We have all heard the phrase *"work-life balance"*, but the challenge lies in truly living it by finding a rhythm where work and life can coexist in harmony. None of us want to miss out or risk losing our position, so we push forward, often at the expense of our health. I understand this predicament very well; I've lived it myself. The short-term drive for income and security often outweighs the long-term investment in health and happiness. And yet, isn't the wellbeing of humanity itself the most worthwhile investment we could ever make?

I believe the way forward is to redesign how we live and work on this planet. Encouragingly, such shifts are already happening in small but meaningful ways all over the planet. Change does not need to be overwhelming. It simply requires a willingness to rethink priorities and embrace healthier models of living.

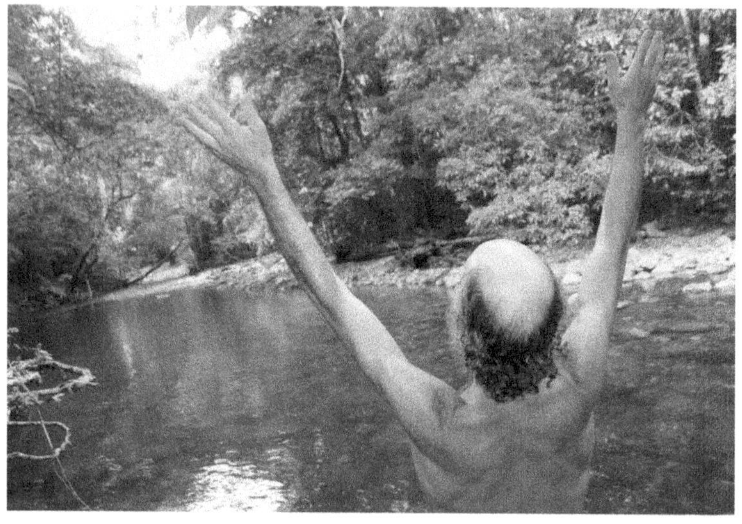

Conclusion

Living a healthy life is, in essence, quite simple. It begins with unlearning the habits that lead to poor health and replacing them with practices that cultivate vitality. By applying the eight fundamental elements of Nature Cure – sun, fresh air, water, living foods, exercise, rest, mental poise, and spinal care – we nourish our cells, keep our bodies flexible and strong, calm our minds, and restore balance when it is needed the most.

Life will always present challenges. Times of illness or injury will come, but with the knowledge of how to assist the body in its repair, these times will become opportunities rather than setbacks. As I learned long ago, theory has its place, but practice is everything. It is through consistent practice that health is built, sustained, and restored.

So, I encourage you to invest in yourself. Allow yourself the gift of gentle, natural, side-effect-free methods that hydrotherapy offers, practiced within the broader context of natural living and healing. There is nothing to lose except the unhelpful habits of the past. And there is everything to gain in the form of vitality, resilience, and joy.

NOW is the best time to begin.

Wishing you strength, clarity, and happiness on your journey to health.

Gerard J. Mifsud
NCP & Hydrotherapist

Appendix

Dialectical Principles

*"Dialectics can be defined as the science of development
and dynamics in nature, society and thought."*
Kenneth S. Jaffrey

Throughout this document I have mentioned a number of dialectical principles which I will summarise here.

1. **Principle**: ***With an increase in quantity there will come about a sudden and dramatic change in quality.*** In matters of health this describes how gradual and incremental changes towards a chosen path accumulate, until you reach a critical point, triggering a radical and fundamental qualitative leap.

2. ***Principle: Conservation of Energy*** – In matters of health this is applied physically, mentally and digestively. Performed during a fasting period.

3. ***Principle: Structure Governs Function*** – The structure/design of anything, determines the function of the said structure. With respect to the human organism, we are designed in such a way that we are herbivorous beings.

4. **Principle: Unity** – Everything is related and correlated, nothing exists in isolation. This is a reminder that I/you are part of the whole and that every part of the body works together for the good of the whole organism.

Glossary of Terms

ACUTE DISEASE: Highly active state of the body's curative processes. This is usually indicated by inflammation and in which the temperature is above the normal of 37°C.

ANABOLISM: A building up process.

BIOLOGICAL: Pertaining to biology, the science of living organisms.

CATABOLISM: A breaking down process.

CATALYST: A substance or influence which accelerates or retards a chemical reaction without changing its own nature.

CHEMICAL REST: Simply means the abstaining of all foods during the technique of fasting.

CHRONIC DISEASE: In the context of natural healing, a chronic disease is one in which the temperature is below the normal of 37°C.

DISEASE: The accumulation of toxic waste matter and obstruction to the flow of life force is the real disease. The word literally means 'lack of comfort'.

HEALING CRISIS (CYCLE) or FEVER: A purely naturopathic term meaning that the body has developed a fever for curative purposes.

NATURE CURE: A philosophy and practice that has been known in the past by various names, including, The Water Cure, Natural Hygiene, Naturopathy, Natural Healing and Natural Living.

NEUTRAL BATH: Normal bath filled at 37°C where the patient lies with head out only usually for 30 minutes to two hours.

PHYSIOLOGICAL REST: Total rest of the body as achieved by using the technique of fasting.

RADIATIONS: The forces of the universe. The movement of radiations is the essence of life.

SITZ/HIP BATH: A receptacle that holds water deep enough to sit in with water to the navel and legs out on the ground.

TOXAEMIA: A poisoned condition of the blood in which it contains poisonous material. The primary cause of all disease.

TOXIN: A poisonous substance which is foreign to the human body and is destructive in its effect, of plant or animal origin.

References

Naturopathic First Aid 1986 by Kenneth S. Jaffrey

Lessons on Health 1984 by Kenneth S. Jaffrey

Dialectics and Health 1987 by Kenneth Jaffrey

Magnetic Waters 2010 by Kevin Hinton

A Lifestyle for Health & Happiness 2010 by Kevin & Katy Hinton

Cosmos, Man and Society 1936 by Edmond Székely

Medicine Tomorrow 1938 by Edmond Székely

The New Science of Healing 1891 by Louis Kuhne

Water and Nature Cure 1955 by C. Leslie Thomson

Nature Doctors 1994 by Friedhelm Kirchfield and Wade Boyle

Wikipedia https://en.wikipedia.org/wiki/Hydrotherapy

Vincent Priessnitz – Founder of Modern Hydrotherapy (1799–1999 200th Birthday Anniversary)

For further reading: https://clinicalgate.com/the-history-of-naturopathic-medicine-the-emergence-and-evolution-of-an-american-school-of-healing/

All of the items referred to in this book, including steam baths, hip and spinal baths, inversion board, and various compresses can be obtained via The International Nature Cure Society website: *www.naturecuresociety.org*

Acknowledgements

I would like to express my heartfelt gratitude to **Donna**, the mother of my children, and to our children **Jared, Laura, and Aiden**, who have been a constant source of love, patience, and inspiration throughout this journey. Your presence in my life has grounded me, challenged me, and reminded me of what truly matters.

My deepest thanks go to my teachers, **Kevin and Katy Hinton**, who not only taught the principles of Natural Living but lived them with integrity, clarity, and compassion. Their example has been as influential as their instruction, and their guidance continues to shape my thinking and practice.

I am also sincerely grateful to my fellow compatriots and colleagues – **Victoria Mohren, Angus Holliday, Matjaz Kovse, Naomi, Saada, and Eric Karlsson** – whose dedication, shared inquiry, and, in particular, Eric Karlsson's research in Europe, proved invaluable to the development of this work.

To the many friends who walk a similar path – **Claudio, Darren, Matt and Marilyn** – your friendship, conversations, and quiet encouragement have been a continual source of inspiration and support.

To all who have shared in this journey in ways large and small, thank you. Each of you has contributed to this work, and to my life, in meaningful and lasting ways.

Testimonial
by K. D. Hinton

I know a man who pushed himself so hard that he literally collapsed. Not once but many times and in different situations. Work, play…it didn't matter, he exhausted himself. His nerve force was depleted.

Of course, he went to the doctor (due to his legal position) and was diagnosed with chronic fatigue syndrome, the symptoms of which include: mental and physical tiredness, memory lapse, lack of concentration, weight loss, mental depression, cognitive difficulties, increased sensitivity to light, sounds and smells, poor muscle tone, headaches and dizziness.

After a long time on the medical treadmill, he decided it was time to do something … something that would give him results. That is, because nothing was working. He just wasn't getting better no matter what he did to improve his condition. And so, he made a decision to stop what he was doing and to follow the principles of Nature Cure.

He left his job and moved from the suburbs in the 'Big Smoke' and travelled to a friend's farm in the far north Queensland tropics. He began a health restoration program, which consisted of REST…physical, mental and digestive, combined with Hydrotherapy, Heliotherapy and Aerotherapy. He ate locally grown produce frugally and slept a great deal.

It's been just over three months now and I'm happy to say that the last time I saw him (we keep in touch via Skype), he was a new man. His skin was golden, smooth and free from blemishes. His eyesight had improved to the point that he wasn't wearing his glasses nearly as much. He was laughing and speaking with a strong voice, his temperature had risen to almost normal, and YES, he was on the road to being *'Born Again'*. Because that's what happens if you give yourself over to nature. It wraps you up in its arms and folds you and coddles you back into health and happiness.

This is a true story. It is ongoing, unfinished, but I believe we can say that the *'corner has been turned'* and the road ahead looks smooth and trouble free.

Kevin D. Hinton M.A. NCP.

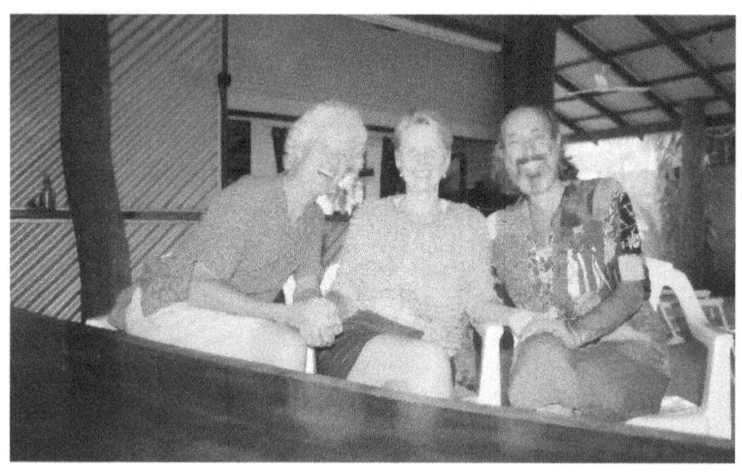

Kevin & Katy Hinton with Gerard Mifsud

Author: Kevin penned these words in 2013, sometime before this book was started. Through the generosity of close friends, I was taken into their rainforest property where all the natural elements required to heal were present. Kevin and Katy visited and we spent time together in the forest living a simple life. Kevin commented back then, "You're looking good mate. What are you going to do now?" Well, the rest is history. Thank you, my friends, the knowledge you have imparted will live on in perpetuity.

Testimonial
by Katy Hinton

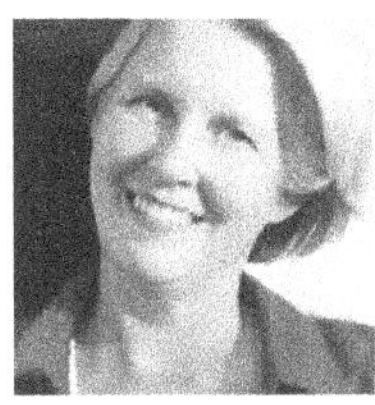

A Journey with Hydrotherapy, written by Gerard Mifsud, is a modern comprehensive guide to the Art and Science of Hydrotherapy. Gerard has shared the principles and practices of water therapy for maximum benefits.

Simply explained and easy to follow applications of water for the maintenance and restoration of health, with only positive side effects.

My personal experiences using Hydrotherapy, and that with patients, has always proved to be a pleasurable and regenerative experience, for physical, mental, and emotional wellbeing. The key I believe, for therapeutic value in most cases, is to apply the practices over an extended period.

When coupled with a Nature Cure Practitioners Diagnosis and Treatment planning, including the basic elements of Natural Living, and Natural Healing, outcomes can be transformative.

Katy Hinton
Nature Cure Practitioner
Magnetic Island, Queensland, Australia

Testimonial
by Aiden Mifsud

A Journey with Hydrotherapy by Gerard Mifsud is a beautifully written and deeply insightful guide that restores a long-forgotten healing art to its rightful place in natural living. With clarity, warmth, and lived experience, Gerard bridges ancient wisdom with practical, modern application, making hydrotherapy both accessible and empowering for the everyday reader.

What makes this book exceptional is its balance of philosophy, history, science, and hands-on guidance. Rather than promising quick fixes, it gently reminds us of the body's innate capacity to heal when supported by natural laws. The author's personal stories and decades of practice bring authenticity and trust, while the step-by-step explanations give readers the confidence to apply these principles safely and thoughtfully.

This book is not only an education – it is an invitation to slow down, reconnect with nature, and take responsibility for one's own health. A must-read for anyone interested in natural healing, Nature Cure, or living a more balanced and vital life.

Aiden Mifsud
Son & Patient
Queensland, Australia

Testimonial

by Eric Karlsson

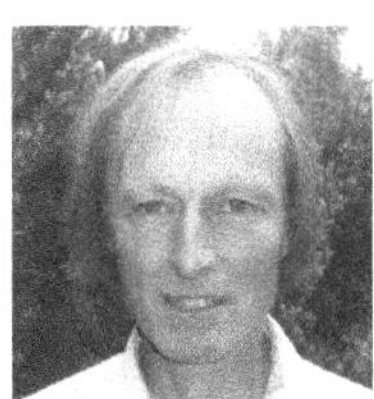

Hydrotherapy is one of the modalities of Nature Cure therapeutics. When the genius and founder of Nature Cure (at the time known as the Water Cure) Vincent Priessnitz first started treating people over 200 years ago he became mostly famous for his Hydrotherapy treatments which did lead to the birth of a very popular international spa movement.

The book goes through the history of Hydrotherapy and describes how to use water as a modality in different ways to maintain health as well as to treat different health problems. Unfortunately, Hydrotherapy is largely forgotten and in very little in use today.

Prof. Hans-Dieter Hentschel (1921–2016) Germany, was a strong proponent of Hydrotherapy and natural healing methods and author of a number of books and articles. When I visited him in Munich 2004, he told me that Hydrotherapy, once used so much in Germany and Europe generally, is now used by only 1% of all Physiotherapists.

The use of drugs has become so much more popular. Regaining our health is not the focus any longer. Big Pharma has made tremendous benefit from that. People´s health would benefit from a renaissance of Hydrotherapy, both as treatment and prevention and leave the toxic drugs with their iatronic side effects, behind as far as possible.

Water is best used holistically together with a healthy lifestyle living in a favourable environment for optimal synergy effect! Sunlight and water simultaneously are a favourite of mine.

The beauty of Hydrotherapy is also that it is available to us all for free or virtually for free. Water is all that is needed for some hydrotherapy treatments. For some modalities, like the spinal bath, a once in a life time investment may be enough.

Perhaps in the near future a renaissance of Hydrotherapy will come.

I wholeheartedly recommend this book as an inspiration and for learning!

Eric Karlsson
Nature Cure Practitioner,
Dr of Naprapathy, Sweden

Testimonial
by Ashley Holliday

The body is self-healing and given the right conditions can heal all manner of illness and accidents. The key here is the right conditions. Sometimes when conditions are not right illness and accident do not heal in a completely renewed manner and leave hardened tissue, stiffness and pain or delayed healing.

Hydrotherapy is a tool we can use to bring the body back to the right conditions for it to heal more fully. Especially when used with the other modalities of Nature Cure.

I have been using Natural Health and Nature Cure as part of my lifestyle since introduced to it by my close friends Kevin and Katy Hinton in 1983. My wife Sue and I have used its principals to raise three children and now they are raising our 4 grandchildren in a similar way.

We have used Hydrotherapy often in this time, on ourselves as well as our children always with the desired result. This is why I can confidently recommend Gerard's book *A Journey with Hydrotherapy*. It is impeccably researched and referenced. In it he tells the history, the reasons and the methods of applying Hydrotherapy.

It is easy to read and understand without unnecessary extra verbiage. Thus, it is not a lengthy volume but succinct and to the point, containing every necessary point for understanding the practice.

It is my hope that Gerard's book can help many more people heal and live more content lives.

Ashley Holliday
Bloomfield, Far North Queensland, Australia.

Testimonial
by Donna Mifsud

I have known Gerard for over 40 years. He is the father of my three children.

When Gerard embrace's something whole heartedly, when he lives and breathes it, his enthusiasm is infectious. Gerard has lived and breathed Hydrotherapy for as long as I have known him. It has been part of both of our journeys to healing and better health.

The knowledge that he imparts in this book is from learned experience and wisdom from his own, very personal health journey.

Hydrotherapy works, plain and simple. I have lived and seen the proof myself and with our children. I hope that as readers of, *A Journey with Hydrotherapy*, that you too embrace the journey to better health and vitality.

Donna Mifsud
Brisbane, Queensland, Australia.

Testimonial
by Matjaž Kovše

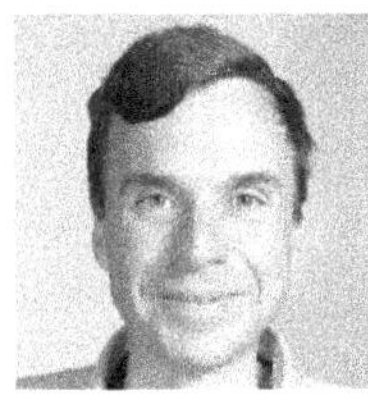

I had the privilege of studying and graduating with Gerard Mifsud in 2014/2015, under the guidance of our teachers, Katy Hinton and Kevin Hinton. Already during our studies, it became clear that, beyond mastering the full art of Nature Cure, Gerard had a particular talent for hydrotherapy - both in its practical application and in his ability to explain it in a simple and accessible way.

I am therefore very grateful that his book is now available to a wider audience. As clearly explained in the book, hydrotherapy lies at the very root of the art of Nature Cure, yet it is often misunderstood and wrongly applied outside our field, especially within medical and alternative health systems. At the core of this misunderstanding is a fundamentally different approach to fever.

The book is written from the perspective of modern people, while carrying the spirit and wisdom of the great authors of the Nature Cure movement of the 19th and 20th centuries. It brings together solid theoretical foundations with clear explanations, practical instructions, and helpful photographs that illustrate the applications with clarity and confidence.

I am sure it will earn a special place in my collection of health books, alongside my most dear and esteemed authors. I hope it will reach health enthusiasts and those who strive for vigorous health and natural solutions, and that it may be a sign of the dawn of a revival of Nature Cure.

Matjaž Kovše
Certified Nature Cure Practitioner
Slovenia & Austria

Testimonial
by Swati Dhariwa

This book is a beautiful reminder that the body has an innate wisdom to heal when supported by nature. Through the author's honest and deeply personal journey with hydrotherapy, the reader gains both inspiration and practical insight into the power of water as one of the essential element needed for the body to heal itself. A heartfelt and grounding read for anyone seeking gentle, natural healing.

Swati Dhariwal
Nature Cure Practitioner
Tamil Nardu, India

About the Author

Gerard Mifsud was born into a family of 10 children. Life was full and never boring, from gardening to collecting eggs from their thirty plus chickens to house chores and paper runs with his brothers. As a teenager he discovered motor bikes, fast cars and scuba diving. In his early 20s Gerard moved to far north Queensland with a passion to follow marine biology.

However his love of diving and all things ocean made him change his mind and he became a volunteer with the GBRMPA and AIMS, so he could spend his spare time under water and not in a laboratory.

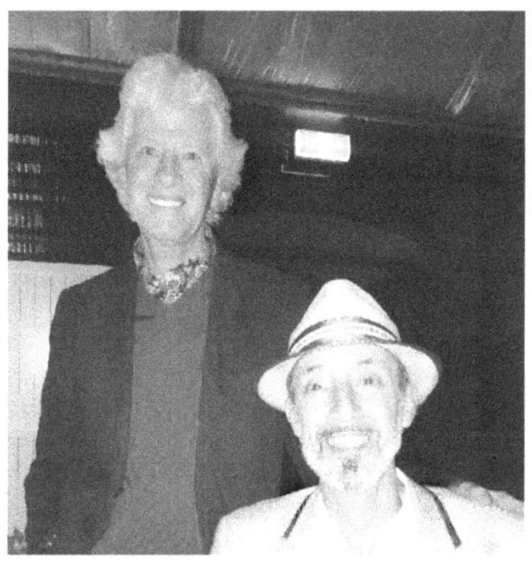

Gerard Mifsud with teacher and friend Kevin Hinton 2017

Gerard discovered Nature Cure through an Adult Education Course at TAFE (Technical and Further Education) Townsville and thus began his journey to better health and his more than forty-year friendship with Kevin and Catherine Hinton, his mentors and close friends.

Gerard has three adult children. A natural entrepreneur, Gerard had numerous successful businesses over the years along with being in the corporate world in publishing and print media. There were always more than a few 'balls' that Gerard juggled… family, home, work, business and life in general. Gerard's children were brought up to appreciate and understand the philosophy and principles of Nature Cure. He always had one foot in nature, whether it be diving under the ocean or the family vegetable garden (and yes there were chickens).

Living the corporate life that was constantly driven by sales, results and performance, eventually took its toll on Gerard's health…. and so, he returned to far north Queensland to begin his *health restoration program* (as his mentor Kevin Hinton quoted in his testimonial).

He currently lives in far north Queensland, where he lives in a tropical paradise. Of course, water therapy is a daily part of his life, along with writing, gardening, swimming, friends and family.